UNHAPPY CHILDREN

UNHAPPY CHILDREN

Reasons and Remedies

HEATHER SMITH

Free Association Books / London / New York

Published in 1995 by
Free Association Books Ltd
Omnibus Business Centre
39–41 North Road
London N7 9DP
and 70 Washington Square South,
New York, NY 10012-1091

99 98 97 96 95
5   4   3   2   1

ISBN 1 85343 308 X hardback

A CIP catalogue record for this book is available
from the British Library

Typeset from the author's disk in Iowan Old Style
Designed and produced for Free Association Books Ltd
by Chase Production Services, Chipping Norton, OX7 5QR
Printed in the EC by T J Press, Padstow, England

CONTENTS

ACKNOWLEDGEMENTS

I wish to thank several people who have contributed towards the making of this book. First and most important is my husband, John Smith, for his kindness, patience and help with editing this and previous attempts to write an intelligible book. My greatest debt to him is for not losing confidence in the outcome.

I am particularly indebted to Elisabeth James and Pam Firth who read the whole of an earlier text and made many pertinent comments; both gave much appreciated encouragement and support. Warm thanks also to Marion Bennathan, Madge Bray, Branwyn Lucas, Bridget Penhale, Dan Smith and Tim Smith, all of whom read parts of earlier drafts, and to Martin Smith for initial instruction to an unpromising beginner in word processing. I am grateful to my publisher, Gill Davies, for her friendliness and help to a first-time author.

Two institutions have greatly assisted my work: at the beginning of the project various members at the Woodrow Wilson International Center for Scholars, Washington D.C., helped in innumerable ways during a six-month stay when my husband was a Research Fellow and since my return to England the staff of the library at the National Children's Bureau have never failed to give willing help over a number of years. I am grateful to both organizations.

On a more personal level, the book would not have been written without the forbearance of my three sons Dan, Martin and Tim while they were growing up. They taught me a great deal, not least that parenting can be interesting, enjoyable and rewarding – for much of the time at least. I trust they do not see themselves as subjects of a book with this title.

During the years many children and parents have shared their unhappiness with me; for this I feel greatly privileged and indebted to them all. My thanks go to the many colleagues, too numerous to mention by name, in several Child and Family Clinics who, throughout the years, have shared their expertise with me and given friendship and support.

TO JOHN

INTRODUCTION

In the labyrinth of theories about child-rearing it is difficult to find an approach based on informed balanced judgement. Previous ideas soon become outdated and ridiculed. This book presents a possible path out of the maze and it is intended for all who have contact with children in a professional capacity, although parents, too, may find it helpful.

A reader may wonder if anything new can be said about growing up and the problems it brings. Two reasons can be offered for adding to the number of such publications. Firstly, it stems from my experience of working with children and their parents for more than twenty-five years, in the course of which I have been asked many times by professional workers, students and parents to recommend books about children's emotional problems. Secondly, it is written with two important Government initiatives in mind. The UN Convention on the Rights of the Child (signed by the UK Government in 1991) stresses non-discrimination, acting in children's best interests and listening to their views. The Children Act 1989 states that the child's welfare must be paramount and the wishes and feelings of the child ascertained; and, further, that the Court should consider, among other things, the emotional needs of the child.

Children discussed here have unmet emotional needs or have experienced trauma or stress – some of a serious nature, others less so. What follows will help to identify such problems and to suggest solutions.

The Basic Theory and Approach

Childhood suffering is widespread and it is hard for many children to accept that, despite their experiences, they are not loved or wanted. Because children's resilience is great, adults can have difficulty in appreciating their despair. Among the unhappy children will be some of the 10,000 who attempt to ring Childline each day; the one in four who live in poor families; the 50,000 on the Child Abuse Register and the 3,000 seriously injured by parents each year. In addition, an unknown number of children are emotionally abused or not valued by their family.

In outline, the theory at the heart of this book is that children have needs which, if not met, cause unhappiness. This distress is manifested by a variety of symptoms including anti-social acts, aggression, anxiety, depression and other behaviour which cause concern. The thread running through, therefore, is a question: what are the unmet needs of the child which cause distress? These needs are identified and discussed under six headings: love; respect; time given by adults; stability; parents in charge; help in developing maturity. A second question follows on this, relating to whatever is causing concern: what might improve the child's and the parent's ways of thinking about themselves and their situation and thus lead to changes in behaviour?

Emotional and behavioural problems are discussed from the point of view of children up to the age of twelve, as well as that of the parents and the family. Sometimes more attention is paid to the child, and sometimes to the adult. The two interlock, each reacting on the other. A distinctive feature of the book is the incorporation of the child's perspective as well as the parent's.

Children's difficulties are a continuum: at one end are children whose unhappiness is so crippling that it affects their development and life overall; at the other, are those whose unhappiness is not so pervasive and at times can be forgotten, but nevertheless needs to be addressed if the child is to grow well. With the exception of very damaged children who need special provision, the book includes the whole spectrum.

In no way do I subscribe to the belief that parents are to blame. Those who might be open to criticism are also likely to have unmet needs and are attempting to solve their problems in the best way they know, given their resources. Generally, they do their best. Neither is it a blueprint for parenting. Instead the basic message to parents is: if what you are doing works, OK; if it doesn't, make changes. Here, some possible changes are put forward.

Theory is treated only insofar as it illustrates a specific idea or makes a child's behaviour more intelligible. References at the end of the book enable readers to pursue topics further.

Without wishing to underestimate research, I do not subscribe to the view that what cannot be proved is of no value. We must look for explanations which fit as many of the facts as possible. In this book the reader will find, instead of mystique and jargon, a belief that many people, adults and children alike, benefit from having somebody's time and concern to help them think aloud in order to understand why they are feeling and behaving as they are, as well as the effect they may be having on other people. Experiencing a caring supportive relationship can increase self-esteem and give the confidence to respond in a different and more positive way to stress, thereby changing behaviour.

The reader will not find techniques based on one specific school of thought, although there is a general acceptance of what Hoghughi (1988) called talking therapy. This does not mean discussing feelings in the light of intellectual concepts and basing explanations on them; instead, the emphasis is on listening sensitively. The efficacy of this approach is hard to prove, but the empirical evidence strongly supports the view that not a few children are helped.

Brief Outline

The focus is on troubled children as identified by symptoms broadly called anxiety or conduct disorder, as well as children who have experienced emotional abuse or neglect. Only the emotional aspects of physically or sexually abused children are included. Further chapters concerning the child in the family emphasize the complexity of relationships and include such matters as the feelings of those with divorced parents, the issue of controlling children, and a personal approach to counselling children in families and individually.

Limitations

The book does not profess to be comprehensive. Some problems have been omitted almost entirely, notably those relating to physical and mental handicaps, and the difficulties of children in care. Children from ethnic minorities are also ignored; this I regret because there is much to understand about the richness, as well as the problems, of belonging to two cultures. Books about these matters have been written by people who have more experience of them, hence they are better left out.

Vocabulary

All books about parents and children have problems with vocabulary. Which word is best to denote the person who has primary care of the child? 'Carer' sounds too impersonal and since the majority of children (about 80 per cent) are cared for by their mother, mother is the word I use, while appreciating that now, as in the past, a substantial number of children are brought up by other relatives, including fathers. Linked to this is the use of the word 'family'. Here it means no more than the unit in which the child lives; this may include one or both parents, siblings, extended family, step relatives and so on. There are many permutations.

The next problem is how to refer to children, there being no pronoun which covers boy and girl. 'She' and 'her' are used to refer to both sexes except where the behaviour described is more characteristic of boys. What to call those who are concerned to help troubled children and their families also requires thought; they may be counsellors, therapists, social workers, psychologists, psychiatrists, pastoral carers, health visitors or others working in the medical, educational or religious fields. With some reservations, I have used 'counsellor' as being the most general term.

As the book presents a personal approach, many sentences could start with phrases such as: 'In my opinion ...' or, 'I believe ...', but, since this would be repetitious and irritating to the reader, it must be taken for granted. Over time, though, it becomes difficult to distinguish what has been learnt by experience from what has been absorbed from others. It may be that some sources have long been forgotten, and if they are not acknowledged it is unintentional.

What follows represents one way among many of looking at children with difficulties or in stressful situations. In the interests of confidentiality, names have been changed and family circumstances disguised.

Assumptions

Some assumptions are made. Firstly, many factors contribute to a child's personality and development, but emotional well-being is greatly influenced by the child's early experience. [1] Even if this has not been satisfactory the situation is not unchangeable provided circumstances alter. Caring relationships can help children change their image of themselves and give hope.

Secondly, parents who feel valued and part of society, not alienated from it, and who live satisfying lives free from the stresses of mere survival will more easily be able to meet their children's needs and provide a loving environment for them in which to grow well.

A Reminder

Inevitably, a book about childhood distress or working with troubled families emphasizes areas which cause concern, but not all children experience unmanageable stress following the traumas described. Nevertheless, the general thesis remains true that unhappiness dominates many children's lives.

INTRODUCTION

Human behaviour is highly complex and many disciplines contribute to our understanding. There is much to learn and much can be understood by being aware of the child's point of view.

The Aim

The overall aim is to suggest a framework for professional workers to adopt, modify or reject, and to make a small contribution towards helping families bring up children to be happy, confident adults. If, in addition, the book can help to make this task enjoyable and satisfying for all the family, and reduce the number of unhappy children, it will have succeeded.

1 THE EMOTIONAL NEEDS OF CHILDREN: THE THEORY

How do we identify those actions of children which should give cause for concern? They have a number of ways of showing all is not well: some cry, some are depressed and anxious, yet others are aggressive, non-cooperative or delinquent. Development may be delayed, or regression and unaccountable changes in attitude may occur. Sometimes there are physical symptoms affecting sleep or causing psychosomatic pain or, more significantly, failure to thrive where there is no medical cause. All point to a child who is troubled.

Problems may be carried over into school, revealed by difficulties in concentrating or underfunctioning. Disruptive behaviour can be the desperate cry of a child lost in a large group of thirty children, saying: What about me? On the other hand some children are adept at separating home from school and it can be the one part of life where the child feels safe, happy and proficient.

What children say about the situation is not always reliable. The very young do not have the vocabulary and believe that they made things happen; they are omnipotent. Older children may be too frightened of the consequences to say anything; others are aware that the adults in their world are so preoccupied that they do not want to know. One reaction is to keep silent and hope things will improve, another is to believe that all children go through these experiences. It follows that adults cannot always know by direct observation that the child is distressed unless they learn to interpret the child's signals sensitively.

One way of looking at the problem by analogy is to see the child as embarking on a journey which could take different directions depending on what happens.[1] What is lacking in this view is recognition of a two-way process, with the child moulding events as well as being influenced by them. From the beginning the infant's personality and interaction with, first, her mother and then her family, affect them all.

CHILDREN'S EMOTIONAL NEEDS

Children have specific needs which are modified according to their age and development.[2] If these are consistently not met the child will react in a way not approved of by her carers, one which may well relate to what is lacking. An emotionally-deprived child may steal sweets or become a magpie, taking things of no conceivable use to her in an attempt to comfort herself; One who is physically abused may be aggressive to younger children; an angry child who turns the anger inwards may use her body to express feelings by tearing out hair or mutilating herself. An even more distressed child can fail to take care and risk being run over or threaten her life in some other way. All are attempting to deal with an unmet psychological need, for the behaviour is the child's way of trying to solve her problem by filling the emptiness inside her or somehow finding self-worth.

Before any effective intervention is possible the first step towards enabling a child to grow well is to identify what is missing. The basic needs can be identified, though it should be stated clearly that in finding solutions, perfection is definitely not the aim. The phrase 'good-enough parenting' cannot be bettered.

SIX EMOTIONAL NEEDS

Unconditional Love

This will be expressed in different ways dependent upon age, but the message the child wants to hear is: 'I'm glad you are around; you are special and I value your individuality.'[3]

A baby needs unconditional love and concern, with its signals being understood and acted on, in an empathetic way. This experience of being loved and having someone to love is fundamental for good growth. Older children, too, want to feel loved, and not only when they are good. In other words, love is not conditional on behaviour, but encompasses the whole of a person – the strengths and weaknesses, the 'good' and the 'bad'.

Respect for the Child's Personality

All children want their feelings to be respected, so to accuse them of being stupid/stubborn/lazy/babyish or bad, or to use any other negative label, is not helpful. Respect means that feelings such as sadness, anger, anxiety and fear are not denied, belittled or ignored, and signs of physical maturity, especially at the onset of adolescence, are dealt with sympathetically.

Children who are respected know from experience that everything about them is of concern to their parents. They are not compared to their detriment with their siblings or treated unfavourably in the family. Statements like: 'He's the naughty one of the family', or 'They're as different as chalk and cheese, are unhelpful'. First and foremost, children who are shown respect receive approval for what they are (their personality) as well as for what they do (their achievements). 'Bad' children lack confidence.

Communication needs to be be warm and honest, without negative comments and destructive criticism. Children wish to be spoken to in a pleasant manner, with the adult showing interest, concern and pleasure. Questions usually need the straightforward answers necessary for the child to develop trust. It is not helpful for an action to be greeted with amusement today and anger tomorrow, and teasing a child can never be justified.

Time From Adults

Usually it is better if parents give time to children but sometimes relatives, friends or carers can help to meet this need. Obviously there is not a set number of hours to give to a child, the time is dependent on the life-style of the family, the parents' personality and the child's individuality. Nevertheless, all need frequent child-focused attention.

Close physical contact – involving touch and being held – is essential for well-being, especially when the child is young, but older children, too, need the reassurance of a cuddle, especially when upset or at bedtime. Talking and listening which include teaching, learning, sharing and understanding, are important parts of good parenting, and time spent in discussing difficulties is usually rewarding. However, that does not mean the adult firing questions at the child, giving advice or asking why she did what she did.

A child benefits from some individual attention whatever the size of the family. Children not supervised by adults for long periods are at risk of committing antisocial acts, and long-term hurt can result if young children are left in the house alone.

Time from adults which involves activities is necessary to provide stimulus, new experiences and challenges. Another important activity is child-directed play, whether constructive or imaginative. The child wants to know that for the parents, too, playing is enjoyable and that they, as well as the child, are pleased to be part of this close relationship.

Stability

The essence of this need, in the words of Dr Kellmer Pringle (1975) is that a child should have a 'continuous reliable loving relationship from birth onwards'. Stability helps the child develop trust in adults, enabling her to be confident that her interests and welfare are safely taken care of.

In a stable family the child can predict events and have a good idea of the consequences of her actions. This is one way of lessening anxiety. Too many changes are not helpful because familiar routines and expectations give security. Children facing major changes, especially those likely to be traumatic, such as parents' separation, hospitalization or an impending death, need sympathetic preparation. How this is done will take into consideration the child's age and personality, but should include the reasons for the changes and their likely consequences for the child.

For the majority of children a stable family gives an identity; this can be positive (we're OK) or negative (we're scruff, no-hopers). The children's attitude to themselves can mirror the image of their family. A harmonious caring family provides a base from which the child can physically explore with confidence, knowing there is a secure place to return to; later the explorations will include ideas and emotions.

Discordant families, whose members normally relate to each other with hostility, militate against good development and future happiness. Marital disharmony, especially, can cause great conflict and sadness for the child and, unless parents address the problem, the tension is likely to be harmful. Antagonism or violence which they witness, although not directed specifically at them, is also likely to affect their self-confidence and be detrimental to future relationships.

Stability implies that parents react in a more or less predictable way. Children with a parent who constantly alternates between uncontrolled anger and guilt-ridden love are vulnerable.

A stable two-parent family is one in which parents support each other and have worked out their relationship satisfactorily so that they do not use the child to meet their own emotional needs. In other words, generational boundaries are not crossed, and children do not have power which properly belongs to parents.

Parents in Charge

Parents have to be emotionally stronger than children and able to make important decisions when necessary. This involves setting limits in ways which are not repressive or unpleasant. Control by fear or pain, humiliation or deprivation, threats or repeated verbal abuse can be damaging because they do not respect the personality of the child. Sometimes parents have to disapprove strongly of behaviour which is hurtful, harmful and dangerous, such as bullying, throwing stones, damaging property, and so on. Some behaviour should not be ignored; some orders are not open to negotiation. This does not mean parents have to be oppressive tyrants. The emphasis must be on attention for approved behaviour rather than a negative response to unacceptable behaviour. The number of positive approving comments made each day should greatly outweigh any critical remarks or orders. This way the child will want to please. It is a bonus if parents are interesting and fun as well as in charge.

Children want parents who are friendly but not a friend – distant enough to respect their growing independence, but certainly not indifferent. This means encouraging autonomy without ignoring their need for dependence. Rigid rules and inflexible attitudes are not required. The child needs to feel that home is different from other places and her family can tolerate regressive behaviour at times of stress. [4] An inappropriate sense of gratitude (you should be thankful we care for you and don't put you in a Home) and guilt (you will drive me away, you make Mummy sad) are unwanted burdens.

Help in Developing Maturity

Children need guidance in learning social skills such as giving and taking, co-operation, relating to others, developing friendships and dealing with conflict in an acceptable way. This requires praise and encouragement for their attempts to please, and setting a few important limits. A further aspect is learning to ask for what is wanted in a way likely to have a successful outcome. In this way immediate gratification will be modified. Children should have responsibility and some areas of control dependent upon their age, personality and maturity. To know that others rely on them is an important lesson and making decisions, however small, helps to develop self-esteem.

To grow well the child has to have good adult models to copy: models of acceptable behaviour and responsible attitudes to honesty, integrity and co-operation; concern for the less fortunate members of society such as the old and disabled; and tolerance for minorities. All these need to be inculcated by example. Parents' degree of control and method of dealing with conflict are especially important in providing acceptable patterns for their children to emulate. By experiencing warmth and concern themselves, children learn to feel sympathy for others and to value their difference.

Morality is learnt mainly (but not exclusively) by observing the actions of those they love and trust.

Children thrive on opportunities to use their ability, creativity and initiative. The pursuit of excellence is a desirable goal, whether for themselves or their group, providing winning does not become an end in itself to be achieved at all cost.

The opportunity to be alone, providing a time when feelings and thoughts can be explored, experiences absorbed and ideas developed, should not be forgotten. If increasing independence and growth is welcome and enjoyed by caring adults, then children will be more inclined to look forward to the next stage of development with pleasure.

PERFECTION IS IMPOSSIBLE!

Parents cannot possibly meet all their children's needs all the time. They have important needs of their own to consider and all have their share of ordinary human failings. What has been offered here is a checklist which, if there are difficulties, might indicate areas to be thought about and changed if possible.

2 CHILDREN'S FEARS AND ANXIETIES

Robin was quite often beaten by his father for reasons he did not understand. Being frightened at home, he lived in constant fear of failing to please, but at school he was difficult and aggressive. Harriet had been hurt in a car accident, an event which left her fearful of crossing the road but otherwise with little apparent effect. Glen's house had been burgled and for a time he could not sleep – he was frightened, insisting that all the lights were left on and the windows securely locked. After a time the nightly routine became less compulsive until eventually it was no longer needed.

These three children had all experienced fear – apprehension arising from specific causes – through different circumstances. Robin's fear of his father had developed into an anxiety which permeated other areas of his life, whereas the trauma of the accident still affecting Harriet was contained. Glen's burglary could easily have had long-term consequences if he had not been sympathetically handled.

They illustrate one of the problems in thinking about children's fears: the great range in the severity of the experiences and the tremendous variety in children's reactions. It may be impossible to grow up without some fear and anxiety, which the majority of children are able to overcome so that their overall development is not impaired. It is when the stress is too great and spills over into daily life, or where the children or someone else is troubled by the resulting behaviour, that some intervention is needed.

The child's response to a fearful event is often temporary and dealt with by parents and others who are concerned, but sometimes it gives rise to anxiety – a more generalised apprehension about future events, which leaves the child troubled, miserable or wretched; in other words an unhappy child. It is therefore essential to consider children's fears, bearing in mind that many of them are temporary and universal. There should be concern when specific fears, because of their nature or the way they are handled (or ignored), become pervasive anxieties which dominate the lives of children, causing them constant apprehension about what might happen in the future and maybe leading to obsessional behaviour. A troubled mind detracts from good development in many areas of life.

Some, with less severe problems, have good experiences which counter the anxiety and leave them with enough emotional energy to develop reasonably well, especially if they find someone who respects their feelings.

One difficulty is to know just when anxiety is playing a large part in a child's inner world because, for many reasons, it is often impossible for the child to share her feelings. Rather, she hopes that adults will pick up clues from her behaviour that something is amiss. The extent of childhood anxiety is considerable [1] and the importance of early intervention irrefutable.

BABIES' FEARS AND ANXIETIES

A baby responds to a smiling face by smiling. The face responds; the baby has made it happen. The message she receives is: I have some control and because you look at me with warmth and affection, you hold me and keep me safe and (usually) know what I need, then I feel valued and therefore value myself. Because I am not anxious I can concentrate on learning and growing. I am all right. If the face does not respond the baby becomes anxious and a little self-esteem is lost.

Small babies are frightened of many things but possibly what is most important is the fear of being abandoned, much in evidence around six months and continuing well into the second year. This fear has been observed in children of many different cultures and is probably universal. Infants having to accept that the mother is not available all the time deal with this unpalatable truth by having a comforter. Called by Donald Winnicott (1958) a 'transitional object', it is a symbol, an illusion related to both the inner world of the child and exterior reality. Another way babies relieve tension is by sucking the thumb or fingers, especially on going to sleep, when anxiety appears to be greatest. For good mental health, most, though by no means all, need such aids for comfort and as a link to a loving mother; the child is depending on its own resources.

Crying

Many healthy babies cry a lot for no apparent reason but there are many obvious physical causes for a baby's crying, such as hunger, colic, wind, teething, infection and pain. [2] We can surmise, too, that the baby responds to stress in the home. Some are not handled gently enough or are cared for by many different people. Others do not receive enough physical contact – there are indications that babies benefit from being carried around or held. In all these situations, crying is a protest. Babies of depressed mothers, who are often those lacking stimulation, cry to get a reaction from their parent, and this is a healthy protest indicating that some hope remains. By way of contrast, the cry of those who are bounced around and stimulated endlessly is saying: 'Leave me alone!'.

Crying may be experienced by a mother as an attack, a rejection of herself as a mother, undermining her confidence and causing her to feel angry. 'If the child loved me,' she says to herself, 'she wouldn't cry like this and make me feel bad; I won't love it'. The tears remind the mother of herself as a child; unconsciously she feels that they should be her tears shed for herself.

Sleeping

Babies have many different sleep patterns. Some are unpredictable and sensitive by nature and respond to situations with intensity; they are more likely to have difficulty in sleeping than easy-going children. [3] Fussy and irritable babies who are bad sleepers from the start may remain so for some months. This may be a consequence of the child's personality which always has to be considered when tackling sleep problems; to blame parental handling in these circumstances is not relevant or helpful. Nevertheless, parents can contribute to a solution by remaining calm and firm and by helping the growing baby differentiate between night and day. At first they may need to reassure by their presence, talking softly, but should not pick up the child or provide any stimulation. To change the pattern might take a little while but in the end everyone will benefit.

Problems in getting a small child to go to sleep and then to stay asleep through the night can be among the worst that parents encounter. [4] Their own tiredness and desperation add to the problem and make it more difficult to see a solution. Parents' guilt and fear of losing control exacerbate the tension and add to the child's anxiety which may be hidden by excitement. She wonders what has happened to the strong parents who keep her safe. Why has she acquired the power to make adults so frantic, so helpless? No wonder she is anxious.

EARLY CHILDHOOD

For young children without words to explain or ask questions, and amid so much that is new, fears abound; they may become attached to familiar situations such as having hair washed but, provided they are handled sympathetically, will soon pass. Noise evokes fear, too, whether caused by the vacuum cleaner – that monster in the house that swallows even tiny things and maybe could swallow little children – or by thunder which is more distant but equally frightening for some children because noise is associated with anger.

Fears arise from the growing awareness of being small and not very competent. Adults can't always know what the infant wants, and the resultant frustration causes anger. But to be angry with the person you most need and depend on creates tension and maybe the fear of revenge. It is important for the child to have opportunities for 'kissing better', otherwise fears will emerge, especially at night. Families may need to consider whether there are opportunities for their child to make reparation when appropriate. To express anger and learn to 'make it better' is an important human attribute for everybody, even three-year-olds.

At a time when the wish for independence is great, separation anxieties are also prevalent. Imaginative play is perhaps the most helpful activity for dealing with the fears of young children: they can then be externalized and the fantasy can have a different ending; one over which the child, in imagination, has some control.

A concern about broken things is part of the feeling that everything must be right. The distress if the biscuit is broken or the wheel has come off the toy truck are very familiar to mothers of two- or three-year-olds and can be symbolic of other, more important things getting broken. Those which can't be mended are especially worrying for the child, possibly because they mirror the child's own fragility and powerlessness. And broken things might mean disapproval or punishment.

Food

Feeding is a microcosm of the mother–child relationship. A meal is more than a meal, it is a gift from the mother which, if refused by the child, can arouse her frightening anger and intolerable rejection. For success, empathy is needed to manage sensitive timing. A small child will want, besides eating, to socialize or experiment, neither of them activities welcomed by a fraught mother.

For the child, mealtimes can be a battleground on which, if the parents see it in those terms, they rarely emerge victorious. They might ask themselves whether the battles over other issues are being handled as sympathetically as they might be or whether the enjoyment of eating has been lost sight of. It will be quite impossible for the young child to actually enjoy the beans on toast when her mother is threatening terrible things will happen unless every one is eaten up. The child wonders whether, if she makes enough fuss, she will be given one of those nice new chocolate biscuits instead; any pleasure she might have had in eating the beans has long since vanished.

Children around two and three years old often use mealtimes to be difficult, whether as a way of protesting about a new sibling's closeness to the mother, a response to the mother's pregnancy, or for many other reasons. The small child, skilled in picking up moods and changes, becomes aware of her mother's 'maternal preoccupation' with the forthcoming baby, possibly before she does herself. The mother will be making small moves to distance herself from the toddler – a response to her anxiety about managing two small children. She believes she will find it easier to cope with the new baby if this one grows up. The toddler is well aware of the sensitive areas and feeding is likely to be one in which to protest about forthcoming changes which are causing her anxiety.

Another pattern is that of parents who cannot stop giving food to the child, especially sweets or biscuits; the reasons often lie in their own childhood deprivation, or, on the contrary, in having been over-fed in childhood themselves. Food then becomes symbolic; a kind of obsessional giving related to their own needs and not the child's appetite. The dentists' advice that there should be a least a two-hour gap in the daytime between any meal or snack goes unheard.

Sleep

The two-year-old has developed an identity and can, for example, recognise herself in a mirror, but there is need for reassurance through the familiar, such as hearing the same stories and repeating the same nursery rhymes. Bedtimes can be difficult because the new found 'me' is in danger of disappearing in sleep. Routines lessen the stress. By now the child has a comforting awareness of a sequence, knowing that after a bath there is a story, then a cuddle, then it is time to go to sleep in a bed crowded with three teddies, a toy car, a woolly hat, some Lego and the comforter. Most parents respect these bed-time rituals, and know that for a brief time the toddler is in charge and his illusion of power respected.

Need for Stability

To the toddler even small changes can seem like the end of the world. With so many unknowns, there must be some security and order even if it is the ornaments in the same place, familiar food, 'my cup' and 'my plate'.

There is much to be frightened of, both inside and outside. Inside is the fear that you are a bad child who might be abandoned or not loved: 'Do you love me?' is not an idle question for two- and three-year-olds. Outside there are great big dogs who bite and it is pointless for adults to say there is nothing to worry about when the dog is as big as an elephant, has jaws like a crocodile and makes a noise like thunder. Things which are large and noisy, or unpredictable, make you scared if you are small.

To sort out what is true and what is fantasy can lead to short-term phobias or fears of things which have been harmless in the past; in this magical world anything can happen. Repeatedly asking questions to which the answers are known help you to be sure of something.

Feelings

One problem for the three-year-old is that of both loving and hating the same person because he or she is not exclusively the child's. If the hate is too strong that person may retaliate and do you harm, a risk you cannot take if you are small and your overriding need is to be loved. One way of dealing with the dilemma is to disguise the negative feeling in some way or to put it into someone or something else. Two examples will show how this works.

Jane's mother, preoccupied with her job, caused Jane to feel rejected and angry; Jane, fearful that an outward expression of anger would make things worse for her, unconsciously projected her anger into food provided by her mother. She experienced it as poisonous and as a result would eat very little. In her mind she had lost touch with the warm, nurturing mother that she had experienced before. Meanwhile, her confused mother, feeling attacked and rejected by her 'naughty' daughter, responded aggressively without understanding Jane's distress. They had lost a previously warm relationship and needed mutual understanding to recapture it.

Andrew, upset at the arrival of a new brother, had an imaginary companion to whom he attributed all the naughty angry things he would have liked to have said or done to the new arrival, splitting them off from himself to avoid conflict. Had this continued indefinitely, his future mental adjustment might have been affected.

One view related to what might be seen as a growth of conscience is the development of what has been called an 'inner parent' who is often punitive. Dolls get beaten, teddies thrown into the corner. This phase is accompanied by fears of witches and burglars. If, as has been suggested, the child fears her own destructive powers can harm herself and her loved person, it is no wonder children of this age need reassurance, closeness and cuddles – a view supported by Rutter's research (1992) which indicated the peak prevalence of fears is at about the age of three.

Both these reactions to the fear of reprisal are to some degree necessary for emotional health, but they can also be messages about things not being right for the child and need to be thought about in the context of the whole relationship. Is food one battle among many in Jane's relationship with her mother, or a temporary phase to remind her mother that she is around? Is Andrew able to express his anger in other ways, or is his family unable to tolerate negative feelings? Is the behaviour temporary and related to a change in the family to which the child responds by retreating into an earlier, safer way?

All children show some signs of tension, often expressed by physical symptoms such as nail biting, fidgeting or stammering. With increased maturity, new fears are added to the underlying anxiety about separation. Parents leaving the child with a baby sitter in the evening may have difficulties not previously apparent. Another new feeling is shame: the three-year-old is concerned at being babyish, as, for example, shown by the little boy who had to wear a nappy in hospital following an operation – this was much more distressing for him than the treatment he received.

Parents can be disturbed by behaviour which affects the way the family functions: for instance, a refusal to eat food enjoyed by others. They can be also concerned by behaviour more appropriate to a younger child, signifying distress related to events in the child's life. An obvious example would be a toddler's understandable reversal to clinging behaviour after a stay in hospital.

Anxiety can be triggered by seeing others who have a physical ailment or are different in some way from the people the child knows. Thus, some years ago, a Russian child of about four, who was interviewed on TV, told the reporter she did not like President Gorbachev because, she explained, he has a mark on his head.

Small children are adept at using imaginative play to deal with anxiety. 'My magic sword will kill any dragon', or: 'My crown makes me queen and I will be in control of everybody in the world', they say with courage and conviction. When the father of three small boys gave them balaclava helmets which had 'fallen off the back of a lorry', they fell asleep wearing them, well protected by Daddy's gift that night, despite three sweaty heads.

Uncertainties of another kind arouse anxiety in the child approaching four, who is learning that other parents make different rules and have different values from her own. In this house you can jump on the furniture but not in that one. This family sit at the table until they have finished their meal and expect the children to do so, within reason, but next door they wander around while they eat. These parents mind about children getting dirty, those laugh. Is there no one way which is right? The development of a conscience and a concern about right and wrong can cause anxiety at this age; it is not unknown for four-year-olds to ask for punishment in an attempt to deal with the strong feelings produced by actual wrongdoing or merely wicked thoughts which are still perceived as having almost the same force as deeds.

Such feelings may invade sleep. Although most four-year olds sleep undisturbed, some have a temporary phase of nightmares. They put their heads under the bedcovers because this can be a very frightening time, once the demands of the day come to an end and angry thoughts and frustrations are given expression in night terrors. Pre-school children's fears are often coloured by fantasy which peoples the imagination with demons, bad men and burglars. These are only some of the menacing visitors who torment children when they feel most unprotected, and come to take them away. And, whatever adults say, there are monsters – they come in the night.

Four-year-old Alex could not sleep because monsters came into his room. His parents tried different ways to comfort him, but each night the monsters returned to frighten him. That went on until one night his father opened the window wide and with great conviction told the monsters to fly away for ever. Alex asked if they had gone. 'Yes', said his father, 'they've gone back to where they belong'. 'Good' said Alex, 'now I'm safe', and turned over and immediately went to sleep. That particular fear had been dealt with by a dad who was much more powerful than any number of horrid creatures.

Children's anxiety is often related to harm coming to themselves or to people they care for. Thoughts can be as powerful as words, especially if there is an emotional conflict. The angry feelings have to be kept hidden because of fear of retaliation, but as thoughts might have the power to wound, the child needs to keep an eye on the recipient of her mixed feelings. Suppose, when yesterday she said: 'I wish you were dead', her mother had really died? It would be her fault. But only a very bad child would have such thoughts, so maybe she would be punished anyway; perhaps she herself would die in the night. Life is full of terror. She needs to be constantly on the lookout in case her worst fears are realized.

STARTING SCHOOL

Fears about starting school, even for those whose life has been relatively free from trauma, are possible because they are having to deal with a change from the comparative quiet of home to school, where the bustle and confusion of many children together, and the difficulty of finding a place in a new situation, can be stressful. Separation anxieties and, more specifically, those concerned with being hurt by other children and those relating to going to the lavatory, need to be dealt with sympathetically.

One almost unmentionable experience a small child may have on entering school, and one which both parents and teachers often deny, is that of being bullied by older children. Sometimes an isolated child, brought up without violence, is bullied. Parents are then presented with a dilemma: on the one hand, they do not want their child to be aggressive. On the other, unless the victim is encouraged to be more confident and assertive, school could be an unhappy place for a long time. A few young children do the bullying, sometimes because they have experienced violence at home and sometimes because they lack social skills: children might have no concept of how others feel, and no picture of themselves and the effect of their behaviour on other children.

MIDDLE CHILDHOOD

In middle childhood some fears persist from an earlier age, notably those of fierce or unpredictable animals, or of being abandoned.

Dislike of the dark, which increases a child's sense of smallness and powerlessness, lasts a long time for a great many children. The fear of being physically harmed can denote a deeper anxiety; seven-year-old Nigel was frightened of his house falling down, whereas his twin brother worried about a man getting into the house at night and shooting him; their father had recently left home, leaving both children feeling unsafe. The belief in ghosts and witches has not quite disappeared. Liza, aged seven drew a number of ghosts, explaining that they weren't real but they had chains and they can chase little girls. They disappear when it is light but – and this was a good joke – once, one of them went to school.

Around the age of ten these kind of fears begin to fade, presumably because of the growing sense of reality. Anxieties are increasingly centred round future events, activities or social situations. More tangible fears relate to being different from contemporaries or to being ridiculed. The fear of failure can be considerable, especially for children whose parents have high expectations but do not provide the necessary experience of success and creativity, or who fail to express pleasure in the child's achievements.

OTHER INFLUENCES

Depending on her personality, a child's anxiety may be triggered by a forgotten event which has left an unspecific belief that something terrible is about to happen. It may also be copied through watching the behaviour of a close relative. Such feelings are widespread and not serious unless they have a detrimental effect on the child's development or functioning.

PHYSICAL SIGNS

Anxiety may be expressed by bodily symptoms, including headaches, nausea and stomach pains; they do not have a physical cause but are nonetheless real. They can be brought on in different ways, such as by separation, or anger which cannot be expressed. Sometimes the symptom can be understood in the context of family functioning and relationships. In some families, for example, people only receive attention when they are physically ill.

As with all symptoms, it is worth considering if the child's needs have been fully met. Is she being given enough attention? Could the sleep difficulties be related to wanting more adult time, physical contact or demonstration of love? Is a toddler not clear about what the limits are because they are not clearly defined or communication is confused? Love, respect, adult time, stability, parents in charge, help with maturity – is anything missing?

Enuresis and Encopresis (Wetting and Soiling)

Reasons why young children wet their beds or themselves are legion and it cannot be assumed that emotional problems are present without considering some more obvious questions first. For example, is the child physically developed enough to have control? Eighteen to twenty months old is often suggested as the earliest age to start training, provided the child feels it has some control in the situation and the desire to please is present. Are there too many threats or too much parental anxiety? Are other demands being made on the child? If, for instance, there are battles over food, it is not a good time to attempt toilet training. Is there too much stress on failures, not successes? Does the family Rottweiler sleep in the bathroom? Are the child's feelings being respected? It makes sense to consider management first because it is an easier option.

The problem is widespread.[5] Purely physical causes can be ignored here but should be considered before looking for an emotional cause, as should the fact that it is known to be a symptom commonly shared with a close relative.

Emotional disturbance is frequently linked with enuresis, but could be the consequence rather than the cause of the difficulty. The child becomes distressed because of the wetting and then depressed, without confidence. Children of school age who wet in the daytime as well as at night are more likely to be emotionally disturbed than those who have daytime control. The phrase 'crying with the bladder' – coined by Mildred Creak many years ago – is appropriate for these children. What is making the child unhappy?

Encopresis, too, is a global term covering a number of different patterns which need to be explored after checking for purely physical reasons and giving consideration to managing the symptom. It may be a sign of stress caused by environmental pressures, such as severe discipline, or be related to the child's unmet needs for attention. The mess or chaos may be indicative of the child's inner feelings, or can be a protest about not being given enough independence or choices. This, thinks the child, is one area where she is going to decide; withholding is linked to power. The products of her body are hers. Some children are clinging to babyhood: babies get lots of attention and this is what they do, is a thought they would not be able to put into words.

Another possibility is that trauma, such as the breakup of the family or any sudden change, might delay maturation and lead to constipation, with its message about needing to 'hang on' to something. Smearing is often associated with aggression or a psychological disorder, although this, too, can indicate a child who is not receiving enough care and stimulation.

So many possible causes demand a variety of approaches, starting with the more practical issues. Enlisting the child's co-operation before any changes are made is important, as is addressing the mother's feelings. Perhaps she becomes upset if there is a mess, or she expects failure and conveys this to her child. That she will need to have her confidence built up and her guilt understood is likely. She probably feels that her child is the only one who soils and that she has failed, but if such feelings are acknowledged she is likely to be helpful and supportive and enjoy her child again. The part the father plays and his reactions to the symptom may be a key factor.

When Peter's mother was expecting her second child, she and Peter, aged three, would lie on the bed together having an afternoon rest. Peter enjoyed this closeness with his mother and was excited about the coming baby. 'My baby', he said, but when the baby arrived he found that it wasn't his baby, but his mother's. This realisation coincided with the onset of very severe constipation. His 'baby' was still inside him. Before the symptom cleared up his mother had to give him time and closeness again so that he could feel a loved and valued child. Not only a new baby, but any anxiety the child is experiencing might be significant; a still-birth, parental discord or absence are all possible triggers.

Behaviour modification techniques are often the treatment recommended for these symptoms and, though the fears themselves are left unacknowledged, some children benefit from the extra attention they receive by such programmes, causing a knock-on effect on the pattern of relationships. Because the child is receiving more attention she responds favourably, causing her to be seen more positively by her family. The result is both a gain in confidence which indirectly increases the ability to overcome the original anxiety, and an improvement which benefits the whole family, despite the underlying cause not having been dealt with.

For children under four, encopresis is not seen as a serious problem but if the symptom persists a paediatrician should be consulted to rule out any physical causes. Very occasionally encopresis is an indication of sexual abuse.

DEVELOPMENTAL DELAYS

Delay in reaching age-appropriate levels of behaviour can also have physical causes, such as a degree of learning difficulty or neurological impairment. If these are not present it has to be assumed that the delays result from emotional distress. The signs are sometimes picked up by health visitors and doctors carrying out developmental checks, but unfortunately the gap between such checks is wider than it was and it is often not until children start school that the difficulties become apparent.

In young children, problems in concentration, 'babyish' behaviour and the inability to wait are among the indications that all is not well. Many such children are restless and their behaviour is impulsive and difficult to comprehend, so that they will destroy without reason or hit without provocation. Often they have a mercurial quality about them, one moment crying with frustration; the next, calmly playing with Lego.

Others present a different picture; they watch the world with hostile eyes, unhappy and inhibited, locked in their own world. Nobody can be trusted, they think. Soon, something bad will happen so I'm better off just watching. The teacher or playleader won't want to know me anyway, so I'm not going to risk becoming involved. Their lack of trust affects their personality. It is likely that children as damaged as these have had very few of their emotional needs met. They have not received unconditional love or lived in a caring atmosphere where adults respect them and provide time and stimulation; stability and continuity have been lacking and success is something they have not experienced.

Good infant and nursery schools can make a tremendous difference by involving the parents in the child's progress, and by valuing their knowledge of her and their contribution to her overall development. These young children benefit from positive attention at school where they can experience good physical touch and can 'play their record again'; that is, they can behave like younger children, playing with dolls, sand and water, or pretending to be a baby. A sensitive teacher running a nurture group [6] is needed to verbalize feelings and help them empathize with other children while indicating clearly what is acceptable behaviour. In such a nurturing atmosphere children can flourish and make up for much that they have previously missed. This is one of many circumstances in which a fortunate child can have

– 24 –

her early unsatisfactory start remedied; bad situations need not be irreversible.

The more-disturbed children and their parents will benefit from a proper diagnosis and can be helped by child psychiatrists and clinic social workers, and sometimes psychotherapists and educational or clinical psychologists working together as a team and usually – though less often than formerly – based in a Child and Family Clinic. Family therapy, which focuses on enabling the whole family to question and change their way of relating to each other, is frequently used.

ANXIETY ARISING FROM EXTERNAL EVENTS

Other anxieties can be divided very broadly into three categories: those relating to external events; to the child within the family; and to the child's environment. It goes without saying that there is much overlap and problems in one category affect the others.

Natural disasters (earthquakes or severe storms) or man-made disturbances (war, violence and car or plane accidents) do not have to be experienced directly by the child to be deeply upsetting. The Gulf War, for instance, made many children anxious. Could the Scud missiles reach our house? Could the oil fires burn us? The effect of children on growing up in Belfast amid violence, bombing and riots, or of experiencing the landslide in Aberfan have been vividly recounted. [7]

Children take cues about how to react largely from their parents. The most vulnerable are those whose parents, because of their own reaction or personality, have been unable to be supportive, especially when faced with regressive behaviour. In this connection an understanding of post-traumatic stress disorder, present if a child has been subjected to a markedly distressing experience, is essential. The traumatic event may be re-experienced, sometimes obsessively. Parts can be recalled repeatedly at different time in particular situations, or unconsciously in nightmares; all cause anxiety and distress. Memory failure may be another consequence. There may be numbness or withdrawal from activities previously enjoyed and, if violence caused the stress, recollection may be either symbolic or real, as a victim, or as the aggressor. Sleep disturbances and guilt can follow and activities which evoke memories of the disaster avoided.

Flashbacks may be visual or aural, smells being particularly evocative for children. So much energy may be expended on avoiding any similar ordinary situation. A large dog had put his front paws on Kit's shoulders when she was playing with her ball, causing her to be very frightened despite reassurances that it was a friendly dog who just wanted to play with her. For a long time she would not go out alone and was frightened of even the smallest dog. She had nightmares and constantly worried about a dog biting her. She overcame the fear by being encouraged to talk about it, and progress, through a series of experiences, culminated in her being able to touch a dog again. This was a happy outcome following a fairly minor trauma, but often the child is unable to function as well as previously, or is left with a sense of foreboding. For some, the anxiety becomes attached to something which had no direct bearing on the original disturbance.

ANXIETY AND THE FAMILY

Ongoing situations within the family which cause anxiety are often related to separation, for it is the fear of abandonment that worries small children most.

The seven-year-old standing in a fairly crowded tube train asks his mother if she would cry if he got lost. She replies that she would, and reminds him of a time when they did lose him. He asks how old he was. She turns to her husband and repeats the question. About three, they think, and she starts the tale: 'We were at the seaside and ....'. He has heard it many times before, but she is demonstrating how parents need to be the repository of a child's history that can be repeated, giving depth to life and adding to a sense of identity and security. While the story is being told he stands still between his parents, but when it finishes he breaks away and begins swinging from the central pole in the coach. 'Stop it!', they cry in unison. All is well: the anxiety has passed.

A child's security is threatened if there is reason to fear a parent's death or leaving home. Dave, aged eight, the elder son of parents who were constantly arguing, had a mother who would slam out of the house leaving two fearful children anxiously waiting for her return. He was burdened by the thought that one day she would leave for good. Not trusting his father to care for them, he became preoccupied with memorizing the route to his aunt's house in case he needed to find somewhere safe for his brother and himself to go to. His progress at school suffered.

Parental rows cause children anxiety about being left or somebody being hurt, but it is the feeling of their own powerlessness to stop the anger which is probably most destructive in the long term. They can be upset by living in a hostile environment, even if the aggression is not directed at them, and react with varying degrees of intensity depending on many factors, of which the most important are demonstrations of warmth and the effectiveness of their support network of relatives, friends and teachers.

Those who cannot talk about their worries because there is nobody they trust are less able to deal with them satisfactorily. Reassurance, nagging or dismissal are never helpful. The parent of a child who has not revised for the exam might say: 'I'm sure you will be all right' or: 'Don't be silly', or: 'You always make a worry about things', or: 'Well, you knew the exam was today. You should have worked'. These remarks do no good and may well be a reflection of parental worry, something which does not concern the child at that particular moment. 'When will I ever learn?', thinks the child, 'I shouldn't have said anything; parents make things worse, not better'.

There are those children who cannot voice their fears because they believe they must protect their parents. Margaret's baby sister died from a cot death. Five-year-old Margaret needed to share her sorrow and many questions bothered her, but she remained silent because the parents' grief was so great that she was reluctant to make any demands on them. Too often when there has been a family tragedy the young child is left to make what sense she can of what has happened.

Anxiety can be related to the roles allotted to children: the daughter who is her father's special person to the exclusion of her mother; the boy who is mother's confidante; the girl who has had her confidence undermined by her timid mother who could not tolerate her independence; and the boy who never did well enough at school to please his father, are anxious and angry in differing degrees. All may be both burdened and resentful, despite the power their position might bring.

A marital relationship involving the child may provoke anxiety. Two religious parents, regarding anger as a sin, prided themselves on never having an argument, with the consequence that all the unacknowledged resentment they felt towards each other was put onto their small daughter. Any display of anger, however minor and however appropriate, was immediately dealt with by punishing this confused little girl who turned the anger against herself, using her own body, picking and biting herself until she bled. Her self-inflicted pain was an attempt to reduce the guilt caused by feeling wicked.

A father, unloved as a child, can have difficulty in helping his own child feel valued, thus causing the child to be never quite sure of her parent's reaction; whatever her father's true feelings she does not know whether she is really loved. Such a parent, hiding his lack of understanding and confidence by teasing, may cause the child to grow up lacking self-esteem. This can be the pattern for a child in the family who becomes a repository of guilt, shame or failure for other family members.

Boys, when they are anxious, become particularly adept at concealing fears because it is less acceptable for them to show vulnerability. Aggressive and boastful behaviour, or covering up in a belligerent way, are attempts to hide a very fearful child within. They may bully timid children who are a reminder of this unacceptable part of themselves. Girls can react in this way too, but, equally, may cling and cry, wanting reassurance in order to face any difficulty, however small. Fears relate, more than before, to a greater awareness of danger, which is itself the product of greater independence and mobility. Learning control in the face of anxiety is seen as essential, especially for boys in our culture; crossed fingers or not stepping on the cracks in the pavement are worth a try.

Children who are not loved are prone to fears. They may think that if Mummy and Daddy don't care for you, or obviously prefer your brother, then you must be bad. They react in a variety of ways, the general expectation being that no one will like them, so they behave in ways that will ensure nobody does. Children who haven't given up hope of being loved may have a recurrence of the fear during early childhood that the angry feelings inside them will cause their parent to become ill and maybe die. This intensifies anxiety. It is my wicked thoughts, a child thinks, which are responsible; the accompanying overwhelming guilt making it difficult to separate, develop and grow independently.

Harsh or unsympathetic handling is justified by some parents who think that they are doing what is best. This is the way they were handled and they were not harmed by it, they believe. The children, accepting that parents are good, see themselves as bad; they are to blame, they are guilty. There is a risk that they become burdened with anxiety and low self-esteem which they hide, quite often by aggression, and a parental model is being learned.

Sometimes such children, trying hard to believe that they are special to their parents and fearful of total rejection, put their fears into other situations such as going to school, or they ask for attention by unacceptable behaviour. Any attention, however awful, is better than none. Some are adept at hiding their real feelings and give the impression that they are fine. Others become independent too soon because they have to parent themselves.

Sometimes a child who has had a relatively stress-free childhood becomes anxious. Mandy, who had been 'Daddy's girl', was ten when she started behaving like a much younger child. She developed a fear of being alone and returned to baby behaviour such as sucking her thumb. No longer an independent child, she became miserable and clinging. Her caring parents could not think of an explanation, because the only change in the family had been an apparently innocuous one – an older sister's wedding. Mandy needed time to trust her counsellor before sharing the fear that she was a horrible person whom nobody would ever want to marry; better to stay a child, then at least her father would love her.

ANXIETIES ARISING FROM OUTSIDE THE FAMILY

Children in middle childhood, spending much of their time outside the home and away from the family, may develop anxieties about their relationships with peers and their life at school. Having friends or being in a group are very important, but the child needs to know the areas where it is necessary to be like the others. These could be quite small matters, like collecting the right stickers or enjoying the same sort of music; more subtle is knowing what your peers find funny at this moment, or what you can boast about and what is not approved of. Some children seem to know instinctively these and many other social skills, while others have to learn to take cues from other children if they want to be accepted. Part of the problem is often to persuade parents that what you need is absolutely vital for your survival – even though next month this will have changed.

The child with interests very different from the majority of her age group, or who is markedly more or less intellectually endowed, or who comes from a family with an appreciably different social status, is disadvantaged. While some will be able to deal with this situation and will be accepted because of their personalities, others will feel outcasts – lonely children who receive callous comments from their contemporaries. Their distress may cause them to become school refusers or express their anxiety by physical symptoms.

SEPARATION ANXIETIES – SCHOOL REFUSAL

For children in middle childhood, anxieties centred around going to school can be severe. 'School phobia' is a term sometimes used to refer to this problem, but for the majority this is a misnomer. Here, concentration is on the specific anxieties which cause children to be fearful about going to school and to feel safe only when they are at home. It is a complex matter. The child, the family and the school may all have contributed unwittingly to the problem and all can help towards a solution; co-operation between the three is an essential first step, especially for pre-adolescent school-refusers.

Noise can be a problem for young children at school, as are the unstructured breaktimes; these things upset the more sensitive. When a teacher shouts at the class the child may perceive the reprimand as directed at her alone. Outwardly trivial matters, like a change of teacher or school dinner arrangements, can be major hurdles making it difficult for anxious children.

Certain family patterns underlying school refusal are more apparent than others. One is that the parents themselves had had difficulty in managing the separation from home to school, and consequently believe this behaviour is to be expected. 'I didn't like school, so I don't expect my child to', is a message to the child that she is not really expected to manage the separation, which, of course, she doesn't. Quite often there is an important grandmother in the background and a repeated history of a close tie between mother and daughter in the previous generation. Separation difficulties often carry on through generations and the ambivalence, too, is repeated: 'It's nice to be close to Mum but I also resent not having enough independence'. That is exactly how the child feels.

Sometimes the father has been pushed out from the emotional life of the family. Feeling devalued and useless, he might let other people do what they want while he escapes into work or an activity which takes him out of the house to a place where he has some self-esteem. In doing so, he leaves the ground clear for mother and child to form a collusive relationship which makes it difficult for the child to separate. The mother may opt out of her role as a wife because the maternal role takes all her emotional energy; the child's development then becomes a worry instead of a joy. 'I watch her twenty-four hours a day', said the mother of an eight-year-old. Work to change the pattern has to focus on the marital relationship as well as that of mother and child. This closeness between parent and child can be a result of past anxiety – a difficult birth or a serious illness. The incident is largely forgotten but the anxiety remains and grows. The child is 'special' but is not being allowed to grow independently.

Parents who have had a very strict upbringing may wish to treat their child in a different way, believing that love is enough. The child then lacks any experience either of limits being set or – even more important in a school context – of obeying other people. The result can be difficulty in accepting any constraints or rules, even, in her anxiety, refusing to go to school. Some parents are unable to insist on their child doing anything because they are too depressed or ill to take the necessary steps. The child picks up their ambivalence, being aware that Mum wants her to go to school, but also wants her at home because she is lonely. Each letter to the school explaining about the headache or severe cold is the last, she tells the child – until the next time.

The anxiety can relate to another family member. Neil's mother had a close friend, the same age as herself, who died. She became very frightened of dying herself and wanted Neil at home for company. Unlike her husband, who was unsympathetic about her fears, Neil mirrored his mother's anxiety about her death. His reluctance to go to school spread to a fear of leaving the house. With help from a counsellor and courageous effort from both mother and son, they relinquished their crippling fear of death, and life resumed normally. Here, as often in families, the father's involvement was crucial in breaking the pattern.

Schools where the atmosphere is caring are likely to have fewer school refusers than those where disciplinary issues are all-important. Co-operation with parents (and, in some instances, compromise) may be called for in the short term, but a strategy needs to be worked out for the child to see home and school working together. Teachers do not always appreciate the effort everyone has made to get the school refuser to school, or the demoralising effect of repeated failure for slow learners or poor readers. 'So you've turned up again like a bad penny' was a comment which greeted one child who had, with great courage, managed to return to school after an absence of some weeks. His understandable reaction was to leave the school immediately.

Adult sensitivity, over a child's stripping for showers, or in taking reports of bullying seriously, might be what is needed. Training in social skills can be helpful for children who have difficulty forming relationships, as can expert help used to encourage families to see the problem in a different way and to use their own strengths to change the pattern.

School refusal encompasses many different kinds of behaviour and levels of disturbance in the child, the family and the school. Expert help may be needed to identify the elements which contribute to the problem. To blame parents automatically is quite wrong. There is never one solution to these complex problems and, as always, the child is attempting to solve a problem in the best way it can. It is important to explore other indications of stress which might accompany school refusal, such as disturbed sleep patterns, withdrawal, or worrying thought-disorders, because school refusal might be masking a seriously harmful situation at home. For a very small number of children there may be a physical cause. Persistent pain cannot be presumed to be psychosomatic, or related to not going to school, without a medical diagnosis.

3 SAD CHILDREN

DEPRESSION

Depression is a word used so loosely that it is difficult to comprehend the depth of pain and isolation that depressed children experience. In everyday speech, 'I'm depressed' can mean that today I feel tired and have lost some confidence because things are not going right for me. From experience I expect that very soon I shall bounce back and, with support, feel all right again, hopeful and reasonably cheerful. My 'depression' has passed. What is being discussed here is very different: it is an overwhelming feeling of loneliness and hopelessness experienced by children, many of whom, including the very young, live with extensive hidden pain which expresses itself as depression. Such feelings are often difficult for adults to comprehend; childhood is a happy time – isn't it? Even professional workers (the author included) find it hard to stay with the intense sadness of some children when they talk about their feelings. So often, it is not what has happened, but how the child perceives the situation or explains it to herself which matters.

CAUSES

For a child who has experienced loss, whether of a loved person, a pet or even their own good health, depression and sadness are understandable. Less obvious loss is a change of house or school; the stress felt by some eleven-year-olds at having to leave their junior school, where they felt safe and accepted, can be traumatic. They fear the impersonality of the larger school; the physical size of the older pupils, not knowing where they should be, what teacher they will have next and, most of all, failure because work will be too hard. Sara described it as 'drowning in a sea of blackness', with nobody aware of her panic and fear, nobody hearing her shouts for help. One way of dealing with these feelings is by unacceptable behaviour such as truancy. Another is not to show the distress outwardly but to feel hopeless and worthless; negative thoughts predominate and nothing seems worthwhile.

The loss of a special relationship can lead to the feeling that life is not worth living. Ashley felt like this when his mother became seriously ill and cut herself off from him emotionally. Other children have the same feeling when a much wanted new baby joins the family or when they are treated differently from other children: they don't count; they are nobody. Childhood depression with this trigger is likely to increase because so many children now experience a change in their family life caused by parental separation.

Children whose needs have not been met from an early age, especially those who have been subjected to numerous separations, may have a fundamentally depressed outlook. They have learned very early in life that they were not wanted and presume this was because they were bad: they cause bad things to happen; they expect to fail. This has been referred to by Seligman (1975) as 'learned helplessness' a phrase containing an implied optimism, for what has been learned can presumably be unlearned. It is a useful concept but does not help us understand the depth of loneliness felt by the depressed child.

This depressive state may lie just below the surface, often hidden from others because the child is 'good' and quiet or has social skills which mask true inner feelings. But the intrusive depression is waiting to surface at the next real or imagined hurt, always there, destructive and dangerous, causing suicidal thoughts. The triggers will be remarks which undermine fragile self-esteem or cumulative negative comments and criticisms. When Patrick was born his mother was very disappointed as she was confident he would be a girl – a fact she vehemently denied, although she could not control her teasing comments: 'Crying again? You should have been a girl'; 'Wimp'; 'Sissy'; and 'Wet', were epithets she used frequently. Patrick's father and brothers joined in the attack, increasing his isolation and despair. He felt he could do nothing right and thought that even if he tried to take his own life he would fail. He was a lonely ten-year-old, in an apparently loving, stable family, trying hard to keep his unhappiness a secret. Unless circumstances change for these children, this single fact that they are unloved and unwanted leads to a life-sentence of vulnerability.

SIGNS

Some symptoms of depression are fairly general; first and foremost is the child's demeanour and mood. She looks sad and dejected, lethargic and alone, lacking energy and losing interest in activities which previously were enjoyable. Other signs may be loss of appetite or sleep problems. The ability to make friends is likely to be diminished, in part because the child is no longer fun to be with, in part because she feels different from other children – alienated from them. Thoughts are often confused and it is usually difficult to concentrate, consequently the lack of progress makes the depression worse. One may surmise that a proportion of children who are diagnosed as intellectually retarded suffer from depression.

It is confusing that depression can present quite the opposite appearance. Some who suffer from it are adept at hiding their mental state and are extremely active, lively children who cannot keep still and demand attention, putting up a smokescreen to hide the sadness within themselves. Young children with depressed mothers may try everything to get attention, no matter what; in their attempt to deny their sad feelings they over-react – any attention being better than none – and getting a reaction, however negative, is a sort of confirmation that you are alive.

It is a lonely feeling. 'Nobody can understand', the child thinks, 'and if they could, they'd think I'm mad'. Some children say they feel full of nothing; worthless and hopeless, or each day is a mountain to be climbed or an enemy to beat. In so many situations children put on themselves a burden of guilt for events which, rationally, they could not be responsible for and are unable to find a satisfactory outlet for their anger. Some hurt themselves in an attempt to assuage this feeling of causing harm. Depression and anger (and hence conduct disorders) are closely linked.

Until fairly recently many people thought that pre-teenage children did not experience depression to any extent. This was based in part on the observation that young children do not compare themselves with others and therefore cannot feel inferior. Negative comparison can contribute towards depression. Failure was also not thought to affect a young child, although it has been noticed that children as young as two years old are aware when they have completed a task successfully and know when they have not (Kagan, 1984, p. 127). Repeated unsuccessful experiences affect a child's self-esteem and lead to the expectation of future failure. If this continues children may come to believe that life is not worth living. Various images are used by them to describe these feelings; one child said it was like having to carry a heavy weight which could crush you if you let it go.

SUICIDE?

Many pre-teenage children have suicidal thoughts, although very few actually try to end their life. The younger ones do not appreciate that death is irreversible. Generally, children in middle childhood with pervading thoughts of death feel they can no longer cope with their problems or fears, and attempts at suicide, however minor, can be seen as gestures indicating that something is not right for them. Their behaviour must always be taken seriously.

Four-year-old Clive, the only boy in the family, had a special relationship with his father. When his parents' marriage failed and his father left home he was devastated. He cried a great deal, was irritable and had difficulty sleeping. One day, soon after his father's expected visit had not materialized, he rode his bicycle across a very busy trunk road and was killed. It was an accident, yet this was a very cautious little boy, and for him to behave in such a way was right out of character. Was this a cry of despair, or a small child preoccupied with his sadness and being forgetful? We shall never know.

Another tragedy reported recently in the press also concerned a four-year-old boy, this time one who had been naughty and been sent upstairs and left for an hour. He hanged himself. The coroner recorded a verdict of accidental death saying that he was greatly loved. Again, it is almost unthinkable that a child should resort to such a desperate measure, but what was he thinking? Was this a gesture which was not intended to have such terrible consequences? Probably neither of these children would fully understand that death is for ever.

Teenagers who are suicidal are often lonely children who have usually given thought to what they intend to do. Many of them have displayed conduct disorders, especially truanting (Kahn *et al.* 1981). For some, it seems as if their aggression is re-directed towards themselves. They show their distress in different ways, sleep disturbances or withdrawal from their usual activities being the most usual. Quite often they have given indications of their thoughts, such as giving away prized possessions, but these have not been picked up, leaving family and friends guilty as well as heart-broken.

WHAT CAN HELP?

Children have probably held the same view of themselves for a long time, because depression is related to how past events were interpreted. Anger may be present, but even more fundamental is the fear of being abandoned and lost. If other people have disappeared, so could they. Therapy can enable them to face these overwhelming feelings. They will need to learn new strategies for coping and for expressing these emotions, as well as new ways of seeing themselves in the world. It is all too easy for a child to believe she is not loved because of her own badness, whereas the reality may be that no child would be loved by her family at that particular time. Children may have to learn that to be treated as if they were bad is very different from being bad. Accepting this is the first step towards a child valuing herself.

Parents must be involved because their reaction is important. A depressed child can evoke frustration: 'Why won't you go swimming, you used to be so keen?' says the exasperated parent. Some respond with uncharacteristic toughness: 'You can't watch the telly any more, you must go out with your friends. You're wasting your life. You think you are hard done by but thousands of children are worse off'. It is easy for parents to lose patience after a time and make the situation worse by adding to the child's sense of failure. 'Why don't you snap out of it' they say. 'Why can't you be like your brother? – he's always happy'. Why don't I climb to the top of Everest tomorrow? thinks the child. Parental comments like these imply that the depression is self-imposed. In reality, the last thing the child wants is to be depressed, but the feeling is too strong to deal with alone, without help and support. A change will require other ways of reacting. Depression might help with some problems because not doing things reduces the chance of failure, but there are better ways. The child who appears quite passive is not a leaf being blown about in the wind but rather a person who, with help, can take charge of her life and make choices.

Feelings of parental guilt may get in the way of showing empathy: What have I done wrong to make my child so unresponsive and miserable? Better questions might be: What stops her sharing her feelings? Is there anything in the way she is treated in the family which has led to her feeling that she is worthless and life is not worth living? What is she reacting to? What can be changed? What can I change? Who can help?

BEREAVEMENT

'It was a terrible time when Mum died; I had so many feelings inside me and nobody, absolutely nobody wanted to know. People treated me as if I were an empty shell with an outside but no inside'. This teenage girl, whose mother had been killed in a road accident when the girl was nine, was expressing a major difficulty. It is almost unbearable for adults to appreciate the depth of childhood suffering and this, coupled with their powerlessness because nothing can be done to reverse the situation, all too often leads to their ignoring the child's pain – 'Children don't understand'; 'He's young, he'll get over it'; 'She's playing with her friends; she's all right'; 'Children soon forget'. The reality is likely to be very different but because the way children grieve is different in some respects from adults', the child's feelings are not always appreciated.

It is usual for adults to go through stages of bereavement identified many years ago. Denial is often the first reaction – It's a bad dream, I'll wake up soon. Or there may be a need to search for the dead person. This might be accompanied by many different feelings: Why me? It's not fair; or guilt: – if only I'd ... ; or despair because it is too late to put things right. These are some normal reactions. Anger with the surviving parent for failing to keep the other alive or for having to deal with such an experience, may be directed at something or someone else; the doctor, the hospital, the council or social services are frequently targeted. But, almost as a backdrop, there will be an overwhelming sense of yearning and sadness at having to deal with what seems like an irreconcilable loss. Only when the feelings have been faced can recovery, embodying acceptance, begin and the bereaved person contemplate the future with hope. The sense of loss may last for ever but, with time, the intensity of the pain lessens if the mourning process has been accomplished.

Children's reactions often follow a different pattern. They usually have the same intense feelings but these do not form a progression, so a child might be weeping in absolute despair, but five minutes later will be laughing with her friends. At other times she will be overwhelmed with anger at her inner pain, but before long the anger goes and she will be talking about the future. This may be why children can make comments which at times appear heartless to grieving adults. At a time of great sadness this heartlessness, which is apparent, not real, is hard for adults to take and understanding is necessary to appreciate the reason behind them.

For adults the mourning is like a river moving slowly forward, encountering frequent barriers which slow down but do not stop the journey to the sea. For children the experience is more a series of pools, full of water. For some periods they can be left but at different times each is threatening to overflow and needs attention. This will be considerable at first but will decrease with time, although the pool labelled 'sadness and loss' will never disappear entirely.

REACTION AT DIFFERENT AGES

Young Children

Babies will not have any conception of death, but if their main carer disappears they will feel abandoned. How harmful this is to their future emotional development will be affected largely by their age and the kind of care they subsequently receive. Preschool children are quite likely to blame themselves, believing that Daddy has gone away because they were naughty but he will come back soon. They can feel abandoned and confused, causing their sleep to be affected. Fears abound and some become restless; unable to concentrate as they flit from one thing to another. They show their anxiety by their behaviour, often by doing things conventionally regarded as 'naughty', by attention-seeking, or clinging behaviour.

Children may revert to behaviour more appropriate to a younger age; wetting their beds again, for example, or in a variety of other ways. Some lose their appetite, and some easygoing children become reluctant to share their toys, as if they have to hold on to what they have. It has been noted that children are more likely to fall ill following a death. Quite often this demanding behaviour comes at a difficult time because the adults in the family are grieving for a loved person too and are not as understanding as usual to the demands of an upset young child.

Many well-meaning explanations given to children are unhelpful and add to their confusion. 'Daddy is sleeping', is an obvious comment which can lead to a young child being fearful of going to sleep in case she, too, might die. 'Only old people die', has been known to result in a child's resisting growing up. 'Grandad's gone to Heaven in the sky', is reported to have led to one child being very disappointed when she went on holiday in an aeroplane and didn't see Grandad as expected. 'He was so good the angels wanted him', is another statement which causes difficulty: if I am good will angels take me too? 'Gone to Jesus', is also not problem-free. 'I hate Jesus because he took the person I love,' can be one reaction, 'and why didn't Jesus give him time to say goodbye to me?'.

More helpful might be comments about the loved person not wanting to die but being unable to do anything about it – there was no choice. It might be appropriate to say that most people go to hospital when they are very ill and they get better, but sometimes the doctors and nurses can't make people better, and that is sad. Other children might understand that a grandparent was old and very, very tired and although it was sad for the people left behind, it was all right for him. But if adults don't know the answer to the child's question then the best thing is to say so.

Middle Childhood

The age varies, but it is usually not until children are around five years old that they slowly begin to appreciate that death is permanent, at times indicating that they understand, then making a comment which indicates they have not fully accepted the fact because it is hard to completely relinquish a belief in magic. To understand fully takes a long time. Many believe that one person did the killing; only over time will they will also appreciate that everyone has to die – usually, but not always, when they are old. They also gradually become aware that a dead person no longer needs a body so will not feel cold or be hungry and it cannot move about. Neither does the body have feelings, nor does it feel sad, happy, lonely. Some will be comforted by a religious explanation of Heaven and everlasting life, and others by the notion that it is the loving feelings people have for the loved person which live on. Important feelings are inside people, like a special burning candle which cannot be blown out and will last for ever.

If one parent has died, children may be protective to the remaining one and will deliberately keep their own sadness hidden as a response, in part, to comments about being brave. Boys, especially, are still encouraged not to cry; this is not good for them because the feelings have to surface in some form, perhaps much later. Research has shown that among boys who commit violent acts as teenagers, a proportion much higher than might be expected lost a parent when they were young.

Boys as well as girls need to express their grief openly; this is an important part of the healing process. One child's expression of grief was delayed: Jeremy worried his family because he could not express any sadness and, as far as they knew, never cried after his father's death. Six months later the family dog died. Only following this event did Jeremy's distress come flooding out and for days he could not stop crying.

One problem children in middle childhood are attempting to sort out relates to their ability to affect some things but not others, and to realise that deeds may cause changes but thoughts do not. This does not come overnight, but is important in this context if the child feels guilt through the belief that the loved person died because she was not loving enough or has felt angry or impatient. She sees herself as responsible, perhaps a murderer, and it is this kind of feeling which leads to a sense of badness and of being different; then it is easy to lose self-esteem and become isolated. She has not appreciated that nobody dies because of what someone else thought and even 'I wish you would die' has no effect.

Questions about death become more perplexing when the child begins to realise that it is for ever. They probably have known relatives, friends or neighbours who died, or learnt from mourning dead pets, but 'Are you going to die, Mummy?' hides two unspoken questions: 'If so, who will look after me?', and: 'Will I die?'. Because of their own reluctance to think about death, parents can find it difficult to respond with the seriousness such questions deserve. They may answer untruthfully or give a reassurance which is either a cliché or unaccompanied by explanation, and therefore unhelpful.

Death is often a preoccupation for children in middle childhood. It brings varying degrees of anxiety and leads to questions about the meaning of life in an attempt to understand the finality of death; especially their own death and that of their parents. They are capable of learning that there is no single truth; that people have different beliefs and sometimes nobody knows the answer. Death is both interesting and frightening. To be aware of the uncertainty of life itself is to reach a milestone: the child is struggling with abstract ideas to understand the world and herself.

LONG-TERM EFFECTS

'The centre of me is always and eternally a terrible pain ... it's like a passionate love for a ghost'. Can anything be done to help children not to feel like Bertrand Russell, orphaned as a child?

The long-term effects are influenced by the relationship between the child and the deceased, the reactions of others and what happened at the time of the death. One school of thought held that early loss led fairly directly to adult depression (Bowlby, 1973). This is too negative a view because loss can be countered in several ways. The previous experience of the child (that is, whether his needs have been met); the events around the trauma, such as possible preparation; honest age-appropriate explanations; and loving care and understanding, as well as the quality of the subsequent care, must all play a part in the child's recovery. It is now thought that children who have experienced loss are more vulnerable to adult depression rather than the event directly causing the adult condition.

The relationship between child and parent is usually one of warmth, making grieving straightforward and without the ambivalence that is more likely in adult relationships. If the surviving adult can express feelings openly this is helpful for the child. If she feels understood and not alone, supported by other important people in her world, and they can tolerate her 'bad' behaviour, then the long-term effects are less likely to be damaging. Adults who have recovered well after a parental death when they were children seem to have been given this sort of support and understanding. Conversely those whose grief is not appreciated may feel the relationship they had with the dead person is devalued in others' eyes, causing them frustration and anger.

Nevertheless, all children who have lost a parent can be expected to be unhappy and show some disturbed behaviour in the short term, such as difficulty in concentrating at school or other signs of grief. They may fear dying themselves and often develop fears, especially of losing other members of their family, or the fear of hospitals. Some become very anxious about their own bodies, perhaps becoming worried about being ill or by the sight of blood. Anger, another emotion which arises from helplessness and from many other feelings, is an important part of grieving and may be displaced from its proper object on to someone else.

Because of the nature of this kind of loss and the fear of making things worse for others, children may be reluctant to ask questions which worry them and might be painful for those they would ask. The cry of many unhappy children in diverse situations is: if it affects us, please tell us, then we can understand better.

In time most of these symptoms will diminish or disappear, although a child's sadness at special times – the deceased parent's birthday, anniversaries or Christmas – will last a long time, perhaps many years. At adolescence some bereaved children become depressed if the grieving has not been done satisfactorily.

A pattern which can have negative effects is one in which adult members of the family fail to express grief openly and only the child does so on behalf of all. She fears that the other family members have forgotten the dead person in the course of getting on with their daily lives and gives herself the task, secretly, of keep the memory alive. Sometimes physical symptoms indicate that this is happening.

Just how long the effects of bereavement can last is demonstrated by Mary, whose mother died suddenly when she was six. She had a loving supportive family and appeared to adjust well but the scars remained. She grew up unable to believe that anything good would last, an obsession she managed to hide until she fell in love and wanted to get married. Mary really couldn't believe that she deserved happiness and take such a risk. Counselling helped her link this feeling with her mother's death, which she believed she had caused, and enabled her to cry for the sad little six-year-old who could not talk about her confused feelings with her 'nice' family.

TRAUMA AND BEREAVEMENT

Some children lose a parent through an accident or other terrible event. This is a special kind of loss needing expert help, especially in the extreme case of one parent killing the other.[1] Such children may have conflicting feelings; they need to grieve openly for the lost parent but are likely to develop post trauma stress syndrome (see Chapter 2) and will attempt to avoid thinking about what happened. Recurring dreams and withdrawal symptoms are common. It is only when, with skilled help, the trauma has been faced that mourning for the lost person can start.

WHAT MIGHT HELP?

It is important to find out from the child what she understands before beginning any kind of counselling. All too often we make incorrect assumptions. Those who have a terminally ill parent are often helped by being told there is a possibility of death, and can then start what, many years ago, Lindermann called 'anticipatory mourning', preparing for the event in their own way. This, which is only possible if the adults also have reached the point of acceptance, enables mutual comforting to start before the actual event.

After the death it is most important for the children that adults are honest and open. A tragedy has happened and the children will be grieving as much as the adults, albeit in a different way; both the depth and the different manifestations should be acknowledged. They need to know that it is acceptable to be sad at times and to be encouraged not to forget. This can be done with great sensitivity.[2] Visiting the grave, looking at photographs, remembering special meals or treats are all means of keeping memories alive and are specially important in the early months of grieving. Relatives and friends, or a well-liked teacher may also help, as might other bereaved children.

After trust has been established, some children will be helped by therapeutic play where they can express guilt for what they might have done to hurt their parents, and what they failed to do to please. And they can show their anger, too, if that is one of the emotions the child wants to deal with as well as the tremendous sorrow. This kind of play might be repetitive, the child going over sequences until they are no longer necessary. The counsellor has to stay with the child's pain in a supportive way and and refrain from making reassuring remarks. Neither is it helpful to collude with the child's hope that the loved person will return. Rather, as Clare Winnicott has said, there has to be a readiness and willingness to try to understand even though we don't. Though what is missing cannot be restored, the cry for comfort must be heard.

In this work it is important to help children revive positive memories of the deceased with drawing and stories, but at the same time they may need to be given straightforward explanations to such questions such as what is meant by a funeral; why some bodies are put in the ground and why others are burnt.

An integral part of healing is to express fears and worries about the dead person and about themselves and their own lives. Darren's best friend was killed by a motor bike when he crossed the road without looking. Darren had seen it happen and for weeks kept going over the scene in his mind, torturing himself with 'Why?'. A group of boys had been crossing the road and none of them were being careful. Darren's friend was a very talented musician and everyone said he had a great future – and he was an only child. Why him? 'Why not me? He didn't deserve to die. It's not fair, it's not fair, it's not fair ...'. The scream inside his head was relentless and almost unbearable. An important part of his recovery was to draw his own conception of the event over and over again in minute detail until he could really believe deep inside himself that there is no answer to the 'Why?' question; he didn't cause the death and it wasn't his fault that it happened. Only then could he shed healing tears of sorrow.

Family therapy can also be beneficial to a bereaved family, especially by providing an opportunity for all to share their feelings of sadness and fears for the future. Sharing such pain, whether with families or children alone, is difficult heart-breaking work – for everyone.

Adults often see the dead person in their mind with such clarity, they think that what they are seeing is real. They hear the dead person walking up the path at the time he used to or hear him calling their name. This is a normal part of grieving which happens to children too, but, unless it is understood, can add to their confusion because for them it seems to be evidence that the loved person has not really died.

Children find different means of comforting themselves, often through things associated with the deceased, such as carrying a token of the loved person with them – perhaps something quite small like Daddy's handkerchief or Mummy's bracelet, or it might be a toy that seems to hold special memories. Reminders of special places or shared experiences also give comfort; all are symbols which need to be respected.

The task inherent in all these kinds of healing is to help children keep the memories but let go of the pain. They are resilient and have great powers of recovery but, nevertheless, need warmth, honesty, understanding and, in time, permission to stop grieving and use emotional energy for living their life fully.

4 CONDUCT DISORDER

Conduct disorder may be defined as behaviour, usually aggressive or disruptive, which has been evident over a period of time. At the socially serious end of the scale it includes stealing and destruction but the term embraces behaviour which is not necessarily delinquent, such as impulsive thoughtless acts, disobedience, or what is often referred to as hyperactivity. Difficulties in concentration, being easily distracted and the inability to finish a task may compound the problem.

Disorders of this kind are often thought of as different from emotional distress which is expressed by symptoms denoting anxiety. Yet it is possible to view both as having the same roots, the difference lying in their manifestations. Basically, both are a child's reaction to unmet emotional needs, modified by the unique experience of the individual child within the family, though environmental influences, peer group pressures and social background can play a part. There is never one simple cause.

The evidence, which is rather inconclusive, seems to indicate that conduct disorders are likely to be associated with the degree of warmth and security experienced by the child. If the family pattern is one of hostility, discord, lack of affection and harsh punishment, conduct disorders are likely. Where there is a cluster of adverse circumstances, including a delinquent family member, an unstable family and rejection, the possibility of the child displaying conduct disorder is greatly increased. Nevertheless, positive influences – a caring person who can be someone from outside the family, or a sympathetic supporting school – can reduce the likelihood of such problems, providing they are not too severe.

Children of all ages show their distress by symptoms which are a blend of anxiety and anger. Boys are more likely to express their feelings in an aggressive way, hence 'he' will be used in this chapter. Probably a majority of them commit antisocial acts during middle childhood, many of which are not discovered and are a nuisance rather than seriously delinquent; indeed, in certain social groups such behaviour is culturally accepted and is the norm. Most, with growing maturity, do not continue the pattern into adulthood.

In contrast, deep-seated anger which finds an outlet in delinquency masks fear and hides vulnerability. Many aspects of the child's life can be affected. Poor concentration, for example, leads to slow progress at school (especially in subjects which involve symbols, such as reading or maths) and to a diagnosis of low intelligence which may or may not be correct. Problems with people in authority and sometimes with peer groups are other consequences. Such children are often described as 'easily led' or 'bad', and it is thought that they need punishment to teach them right from wrong.

These children will have unmet needs, but often they will have the experience when young of knowing great fear. This can be of physical pain such as being beaten or harmed by parents or abused in some way, but can also be a mental fear: for example, being shut in a dark place, left alone in a house, or being tortured verbally by threats or fears.

The fear is experienced as terror at first, but as the child grows, so does anger – a healthy step for emotional survival although there is the danger of identifying with the aggressor to hide vulnerability; then he is no longer a victim but a powerful antagonist. For the schoolchild the aggression can be directed at other children, taking the form of bullying; alternatively it can be directed inwards causing them to harm themselves by their actions.

As teenagers the fear which they have successfully hidden behind anger and aggression can lead to destructive antisocial acts involving violence or theft. They may abuse themselves with alcohol or drugs. There are many ways of disguising the basic fear which may be consciously forgotten, but nevertheless remains – insidiously undermining confidence and affecting behaviour. This is rather different from the fairly general 'nuisance' behaviour of many adolescent boys in their search for a new identity and excitement. Girls of this age are more likely to show their distress in promiscuity or self-harm, giving a message of not feeling valued.

IMMATURE CHILDREN

'Immature' is often used to describe a child in a negative way, as if the child is somehow to blame, rather than asking the question: what is causing him to behave like this; what is he reacting to?

A well-adjusted young child on seeing another child crying will first mirror the emotion by crying himself, then, using his own experience, he is likely to give comfort or get help. Later, with the awareness that not only events but other people's reactions have emotional consequences, and if he made the child cry or caused adults to be cross, he may feel shame or sorrow.

In contrast, children displaying what is called immature behaviour appear to be unaware of other people's feelings; they fail to pick up social clues. 'How ever much you tell him off or punish him, it makes no difference; he does the same thing again', say the confused and often desperate parents of these 'stuck' children. Sometimes the difficulties are long standing and can be traced to the early years because of the lack of closeness or failure to have help with mastering social skills.

Harry, aged eight, whose parents had divorced, seldom saw his father who lived abroad. His mother was caring but strict and distant. The father's absence was never talked about, so Harry did what most children do in such circumstances, he blamed himself, believing that it was his behaviour which caused his dad to leave. Missing his father so greatly made him feel both sad and bad. He dealt with these secret feelings by denying them and becoming the class 'clown'. This worked well for a while but the image took over to such an extent that teachers and pupils found him immature and silly. His schoolwork suffered and he became increasingly alone. Had his fantasies and feelings at the loss of his father not been explored, delinquent behaviour could easily have appeared in adolescence.

Aggressive, inattentive children and those with difficulties in control are often not popular with their peers, thus compounding their problem. They interpret the comments and behaviour of others as hostile, thus starting a spiral of negative reactions. A small number respond positively when artificial colouring is removed from their diet, but more do so when help is given with learning social skills or changes are made in parenting practice.

SAM, AN AGGRESSIVE CHILD

For much of his life ten-year-old Sam had caused his mother worry. She believed he was different from her other children because even as a small child he had refused to do what he was told. His mother placated him; otherwise things would get thrown and, later, windows broken and doors kicked. His father had little to do with any of the children except to use corporal punishment, as he put it, to discipline them, and as Sam had no understanding of other people's feelings, 'You wouldn't like it done to you' had no meaning for him.

At first his behaviour was mostly confined to the family but by the age of eight he was in trouble for fighting. The school was sympathetic at first, despite his truancy, because they felt sorry for his very concerned mother, but, after a number of dangerous incidents endangering other children, they lost patience. His mother was heartbroken; she really did love her only son. Her overriding feeling was of failure. She had not wanted to be pregnant when he was conceived but, when he was born, her anger at carrying an unwanted child turned to a mixture of love and guilt. She was the one who had looked after him; it must be her fault that he was such a problem.

Sam's own view of the situation was very different. He loved his dad despite his drinking and violence. He believed without doubt that his dad loved him, though the evidence was weak. Male violence was a more-or-less accepted cultural pattern and if Dad beat him it showed he cared and, despite the trouble he was in, in a funny sort of way it made him feel contained and safe because it established boundaries.

About this time his mother had had enough of her husband's violence and made him leave the house, At first she received most of Sam's anger for not keeping dad at home for now there were no checks on him. One winter's night Sam waited outside his father's usual pub; his father saw him but walked past with his friends, ignoring his son, whose anguish was total.

As a result his behaviour deteriorated and his aggression increased. He would fight even with grown men; they were not his father but served as substitutes. He believed that no one cared for him – even his mother preferred his sisters because they were good – so he cared for nobody, and nobody was ever going to hurt his feelings again. Anger and violence were the ways he hid his hurt, and before long his aggression became delinquent behaviour. Fortunately, he was accepted by one of the few special schools in the country which give children like Sam an opportunity to understand their feelings. He experienced limits which were not based on fear and pain and he gained a self-esteem unrelated to his being the most feared boy in the neighbourhood.

YOUNG CHILDREN AND CONDUCT DISORDERS

As with emotional difficulties (Chapter 2), the indications of later problems are usually present at an early age. [1] Unless something is done, a preschool child who is restless, aggressive or difficult to handle can become an angry, alienated small child in a junior school, finding concentration difficult, falling behind with studies and possibly not averse to taking other people's property in an attempt to relieve feelings of depression or loss. By the time he is a teenager he may become delinquent and turn to burglary, theft or joyriding, and eventually graduate to more serious crime. The case for early intervention is irrefutable, before thoughts and behaviour become dominated by the belief that 'they' are against you and therefore you must get revenge whatever the cost. This is not to say that all children exhibiting conduct disorders at an early age will become adult criminals, but indications are that they are more likely to have difficulties in forming stable relationships or to encounter problems with training and employment. It appears, too, that they are also more likely to become seriously depressed, thereby supporting the view that emotional problems and conduct disorder are linked.

Society can go some way to reducing the number of children whose behaviour is troublesome. Poverty plays an important part because it makes the parental task of meeting the child's emotional needs more difficult. Many children living in poor families do not become delinquent, but those with a double handicap – coming from deprived backgrounds and also being rejected or neglected – are more at risk.

Research has shown that successful development is more likely if children are brought up feeling loved and valued, in a stable home not dominated by discord. It is particularly important that there should be good adult models to emulate, and that the child's environment – home, school and neighbourhood – give hope and a sense of self-esteem. Harsh discipline imposed on eight- and nine-year-olds can be particularly harmful. [2] If early signs of later difficulties are ignored and the opportunity of intervention is lost, the child will face ever worsening problems in learning and behaviour.

STEALING

The mother of a travelling family said: 'The first people the kids learned to steal off were their mothers. The second group they learned to steal off was the schools. Already my eldest son had gone to a detention centre and a borstal. By the time my youngest son was eleven he had had his fingers in my purse and then ripped off the school for £200 worth of sports equipment ...' (*Guardian*, 19 June 1991). Naughty children – or unhappy? Children wanting adventure and excitement or copying the behaviour of those around them? Children from poor families who are isolated from the mainstream of society? Or could the root cause be that they do not have their needs met?

Small children who repeatedly steal money from a parent may be asking for the love and attention they want to be freely given; they fill the emotional emptiness with anger. Taking money is an attack on the parent for making them feel unhappy. Some believe that because their feelings about their parents are so terrible they are themselves guilty and unlovable. All the punishment in the world would not remove such guilt. 'He seems to want you to punish him', parents say, unaware that this is the child's attempt to deal with these guilty feelings. Sometimes parents have to acknowledge their own early deprivation before they can perceive their own children differently, and sometimes their way of handling the problem needs to be changed, and that will involve appreciating that the child is trying to fill an emotional gap in the best way he knows.

Those who steal food may be at least as worrying because what is important to the child is the taking. What has he not been given in the past, or is not given now? It may be love or self-esteem, something he has not given up hope of having. The food he takes is a symbol of what he has lacked. 'Why does he take biscuits when he knows he can have as many as he likes if only he would ask?' say anxious, puzzled parents. What they do not realise is that the important part of the communication is the taking, not being given what is asked for.

Insecure children in middle childhood who lack social skills attempt to buy the friendship they desperately need, even if this means having to steal. Why do they have such a low opinion of themselves? Why do they lack confidence? The problem is likely to be related to the child's image of himself. Those who have been seriously deprived do not develop a sense of themselves as people and, because the concept of people's having boundaries has not been learnt, they would not understand that it is wrong to take other people's things. [3]

BULLYING

Children who are Bullied

Bullying is a phenomenon which parents and teachers alike find hard to acknowledge. It is important for parents to believe that their child is popular and has lots of friends and it is difficult for teachers to accept that the atmosphere in their school is such that some children can terrorize others; both groups have a reason to ignore the problem. Because it is widespread, especially in its less obvious forms, it needs to be discussed at some length; children are more likely to be bullied by being ostracized or by verbal abuse than by physical attacks.

Boys are vulnerable because of the belief that they have to stand on their own two feet or ignore the insults and attacks, so the bullies will pick on someone else. 'You must be doing something', parents and teachers say. Such comments make the child feel isolated at home and at school. It is perhaps because they are less confident, with fewer social skills, and are different in some way, or less likely to be a member of a group, that they make a good target. A small number of children appear to invite aggression although this is a superficial explanation.

'Why didn't you tell us?', parents will ask. Because I could not rely on you to find a helpful solution, the child thinks, and I would lose any control I have over what is happening. Because you feel I should deal with it myself and you can't begin to understand what hell it is. And sometimes I think that whatever makes other boys bully makes you do the same thing to me in a different way. 'I didn't think it would help', says the boy as he turns away.

Observant adults can pick up indications of bullying. A lack of concentration, falling academic levels, coming home late from school, taking a different route home, or a general air of stress and unhappiness may be pointers. Wanting extra money or arriving home very hungry because the bully has taken the packed lunch might be other indications which alert parents. What is not helpful is to dismiss it or tell the child to ignore it. If it has gone on for some time it must be discussed with the school. Despite the level of anxiety which comes to light, it is not helpful for a counsellor or parent to promise not to tell anyone.

As with all behaviour indicating emotional problems, there is no single solution. Individual counselling coupled with help in developing social skills to gain self-esteem provides one approach, for these are often deeply anxious children, hiding inner loneliness by behaviour.

Children who are bullied are usually very distressed because the bullying goes deep into their personalities. They believe that because they are treated like this and have few friends, they are of no value and, like other abused children, are in some way to blame. This low self-esteem may have continued for years and will not easily be forgotten, sometimes surviving into adulthood. Some, in a desperate attempt to find some self-esteem, torment other children; the victim becomes the aggressor.

Children who Bully

Steve's parents were in despair. They felt they had given him a lot of attention and had done their best to be 'good' parents, setting him reasonable limits and taking an interest in his progress at school. They did not want him to be a 'spoilt brat' and would hit him when they thought his behaviour warranted it. They were strongly against cruelty but he had to learn discipline and respect; part of good parenting was to teach these.

When Steve was ten he was in trouble at school for bullying and, at about the same time, had been caught stealing from a local sweet-shop. His parents were devastated. For them, the alternative to their discipline was to set no limits – something they could not do, for child-centred free expression was quite alien to them. What had gone wrong? Was Steve inherently bad? Did they need to be even more strict?

In fact, nobody was to blame. The stealing was a response to Steve's feeling that something in his life was missing, and this turned out to be his parents' approval of him as an individual, not simply for what he did. In family meetings he had been very surprised to learn that they were concerned for his happiness and well-being. In fact, he had been used by his parents to prove to the world that they were good parents and old-fashioned ways were best. The bullying was related to his identification with his family. Physical pain obviously solves problems. My parents hurt me to make me do what they want, therefore I will hurt other children. The difficulties, seen in terms of the family's inability to communicate caring feelings and respect for each other, improved through family meetings.

Steve's parents had not considered ways of controlling him other than physical punishment: they had put their needs to be seen as good parents before Steve's need to be understood, treated with respect, listened to and valued. They did love him but were quite unable to convey their true feelings to him. This was difficult until they gained confidence in themselves as parents and could give up their fear of his becoming out of hand. Only then could they set benign limits which gave security without causing resentment and enjoy having a lively interesting boy in the family.

Children, whether boys or girls, who bully are not sure of themselves; they may be envious of someone or they may have discovered a victim who will provide them with money or material things and who is too terrified to tell anyone. Some will have been bullied by fathers or older brothers. They attract other insecure children who feel safe in a group and can then join in the bullying as a way of protecting themselves from being on the receiving end. Some have strong personalities and are popular with other children. A parent's observation that 'no one will like you if you hurt other children', is often far from the truth. Bullying is a part of the child, not the whole.

Much of the bullying is mental torture rather than physical violence and is more likely to be the action of a group against one child. Victims will be called names or be the butt of jokes. Richard's brother told the children at school that seven-year-old Richard wet his bed. They teased him mercilessly, repeatedly asking him if he had tried the new nappies which were being advertised on TV. In this kind of situation it is easy to forget that all children, both bully and bullied, have a problem. Such unkindness should not be ignored by parents or school. Other children have their property damaged, receive threats, or are ostracized. Because the bully cannot identify with his victim (he wouldn't be a bully if he could), and even though he may have been bullied himself, physical punishment is usually of no avail. If you are hurt by being punished you are more likely to want revenge than to behave differently.

'By my violence you will know me and I will know that I exist' wrote Richard Rollinson (1993), Director, Mulberry Bush School. This quotation may help to understand why some children bully. Violence shows others that the perpetrator is a person who cannot be ignored, somebody who has power and can make things happen.

Such violence can seem to have a life of its own and, without reference to the victim, becomes exciting. The challenge is to help such a child feel empathy for those weaker than himself – no easy task.

Parents who learn that their child is a bully need to listen to the child's version and to convey their disapproval of bullying very strongly. They also need to think what is causing such behaviour. Is he being bullied at home or elsewhere? What is their own attitude to weak and vulnerable people? Is their child demonstrating misplaced anger or having to hide his own fear of being thought 'soft'? What ways could the child suggest to make reparation? It is important to help the victim learn to deal with his situation but even more important for the bully to change his attitude, otherwise he will just find another vulnerable child to bully.

Schools

Schools can help by acknowledging the problem and encouraging discussion among all the children – who may have some ideas about how to eradicate it. Proposals to change pupils' and staff's perception of bullying involve encouraging them to respect each other and require the staff to examine their own attitudes (Tattum and Lane, 1989): anyone who has counselled bullied children knows how much teachers' behaviour influences pupils', and how greatly sarcasm undermines self-esteem. Much can be done by changing the ethos of the school, organising awareness programmes [4] and taking immediate action every time physical or emotional bullying, including ostracizing a child, is discovered.

In 1991 two phone lines were opened by Childline especially for children to talk about bullying; one was in operation for three months and one for six. In all, 12,000 calls were made.[5] It was the extent of the problem which caused surprise and concern. It was estimated that one in five children is either a bully or a victim. Bullying results in many children experiencing years of unhappiness at school and should be considered far more seriously. Those from a different ethnic background are especially vulnerable.

The maxim that any attention is better than none is relevant in this context. What can easily happen is that unacceptable behaviour is rewarded more consistently than acceptable behaviour. The bully gains attention, albeit of a critical and disapproving kind; the victim tells the adults and gets a sympathetic hearing. Both these interventions are important, but attention and acknowledgement must also be given when, for instance, the bully leaves vulnerable children alone or includes them in an activity. Neither should it go unnoticed if the bullied child manages to be friendly, or part of a group, without feeling a victim.

Summary

Several questions need to be addressed concerning bullied children. Why does this child have such a poor image and allow this to happen – does the expectation that he will not be liked come from the family or is there another explanation relating to being different in some way from his peers? Is the problem related to aggression – the child's ability to express his own anger appropriately and to deal effectively with other people's anger? What has stopped him learning the social skills necessary to relate well to other children and make friends? The answers to these questions will influence the interventions needed to change the pattern.

Children who bully raise other questions. What problem is this behaviour attempting to solve? Does the aggression belong elsewhere and is there fear which has to be hidden behind the anger? Has his family experience taught him that violence solves problems, or is aggression associated with masculinity or power? Why has this child failed to empathize with the less robust members of his group?

TRUANCY

Not all children with problems of attendance at school are reacting to fear and anxiety. Many, mainly the older children, have days off school or do not turn up for lessons, but some stay away for long periods and, although this is usually done without parental knowledge, sometimes parents do know what is happening and either condone it or are unable to change the situation. The children, often angry and defiant, can evoke anger and frustration in teachers, and in politicians, too, for they are defying the law of the land.

Truanting children pose the same question as those who bully: what problem are they trying to solve by not going to school? If they are reacting to a lack of appropriate limits then court appearances or suspended sentences can sometimes help, but if truancy relates to a lack of self-esteem and an overwhelming need to be accepted by the peer group who also play truant, such action will seem irrelevant to a child. Some find the school's necessary insistence on order and conformity difficult; others, used to having their own way, prefer to play video games or enjoy the excitement of fruit machines. Some are just too tired to concentrate and dislike having to expose their inadequacies and lack of knowledge in school. Many are unable to leave the stresses of their home life behind. Fear and punishment will be of no avail to most of these children. Attempts to build up their self-esteem have more chance of resulting in a positive outcome. A word of warning, though, may be desirable: self-esteem, which varies according to the group the child is in, has many manifestations and should not be automatically assumed to be at the root of this kind of problem.

Research indicates that truants are more likely to be suffering social disadvantages and be underachieving than those who attend school regularly. These conditions result in their alienation from the school system they see as irrelevant and boring. But the scale of the problem indicates that this is not the only explanation – a proportion of truants enjoy school and have good ability.

In fact, there is a great deal of repetition of received opinions and little proven knowledge about truancy, hence the often-quoted link between crime and truancy cannot be substantiated. We do know that some schools have a better record than others and this is likely to be due to the caring atmosphere within the school and the interest and concern for the pupils shown by staff.

We do not know how typical the case of twelve-year-old Claire is, although girls as well as boys play truant. Her attendance at her comprehensive school was poor from the start, although there hadn't been problems in the junior school. In counselling sessions she described how difficult it had been to settle down in such a big school with constant changes of teacher and classroom. She had not been emotionally ready to make such a change with its implication of growing up, saying she had wished she were Peter Pan. Hiding on the school premises rather than attending lessons was an attempt to protect herself from feelings of inadequacy, but the understandable hostility she received from the staff made her aggressive and defiant, thus compounding the problems of this unhappy, immature, sullen child who had lost all trust in adults. Counselling over one term helped her gain a different image which gave her hope of success; she began to see herself positively, found new friends and her behaviour improved.

ARSON

Sometimes fires can be started by fascinated two- or three-year-olds playing with matches. Many incidents go unreported because parents feel exposure might reflect on the adequacy of their supervision. However, children who become obsessed with fire are in some ways often like those labelled hyperactive: lively, easily distracted and destructive. They may have a high degree of curiosity.[6] Some will be emotionally and physically deprived, full of anger and thoughts of revenge, especially against their mother. Often they have an insecure background and have experienced a lack of basic care or violence in their home.

Insecurity dominates the lives of other firesetters. Three-year-old Kevin started a fire in the airing cupboard where his mother was keeping clothes for the baby expected very shortly. Keith, slightly older, had been attached to his grandparents but had to leave them to go to another town with his mother when she remarried. He felt his roots had been severed and blamed his mother, especially when she had two more children in close succession. Previously he had been caught trying to set the curtains in her bedroom on fire, then later had managed to burn her bed.

Kevin and Keith had both experienced deprivation and rejection, had ambivalent feelings towards their mother and were still hoping to be loved. A small fire would have made them feel less guilty, but the excitement of fire engines roaring down the street and the subsequent attention they received from striking one little match were enjoyable.

In older children, fire-raising may be related to sexuality or to internal problems of control and things getting out of hand; it is a symptom which can indicate a deep-seated disturbance requiring psychiatric help.

CHILDREN WHO HATE

At one end of the spectrum of child-parent relations are children who are loved and secure; at the other end, those who have not had consistent affection when small and grow up hating. They have no warmth for anyone and for them hate is not something which comes and goes but a permanent part of them and their life. Revenge is all-important. Years of being exposed to indifference, inconsistency or physical cruelty have left them without the normal sanctions which modify behaviour. Children want to be loved and to please the person who loves them. Those who have not been involved will hurt and harm, damage and destroy in what to other people seems a mindless and brutal manner.

These impulsive children appear to have an underdeveloped sense of fear arising from the traumas they have experienced in the past. These might have caused neurological changes which in turn affect their behaviour. It has been said that delinquency is a sign of hope in a child; whatever the general truth of this, for boys who hate it is a way of survival apparent by the age of six or seven. Many will have physical defects and educational difficulties; many come from families which include members who behave in a similar way; most are severely emotionally deprived.

Only with difficulty can patterns can be changed for some of these children through altered circumstances or relationships; others require long-term, skilled, professional intervention. It is important for those attempting to help these families and children not to lose hope. Some aspects of the child's situation cannot be changed, some can. Learning a different response is one. If the child is fortunate enough to find someone who will show interest and concern and who is prepared to stand a great deal of testing and rejection, he feels he has some control over his life and consequently some power to make changes.

This is difficult and frustrating work because the child will be adept at projecting his hate into whoever is trying to help, finding vulnerable spots to attack. He may not know any other way of relating to people or perhaps he unconsciously wants someone else to experience the sort of feelings he carries within him all the time. While he is learning to trust, the person helping has to keep caring – and to survive.

AGGRESSIVE FANTASIES

Children's thinking was illuminated by a study of over 2000 stories they told about the drawings they had done.[7] The most violent children told the most violent stories. Children with behaviour disorders were more likely to write stories with themes of conflict, disturbance and anger. The story was likely to end in disaster or hopelessness and the personality of the central character was likely to be a 'baddie' or a victim; both aspects reflect the despair and poor self-image of the child. Aggression, antisocial behaviour or disasters were repeated in a compulsive way without solutions. Especially worrying were those children who talked about everyone dying or the world coming to an end; their hopelessness is likely to be dealt with by future antisocial behaviour or aggression.

Models as well as drawings can reveal these disturbing traits. Dean, a seven-year-old from a disruptive, unsettled home, made models of houses, always in remote places; beautiful and tranquil. He would have a house like that one day and spend his time fishing and caring for animals he had rescued, but towards the end of each session the house was bombed or destroyed by an earthquake. On bad days, not only the house but also the whole world was destroyed by men from another planet. His house was a dream, there was no future and nothing good would ever happen to him.

The study just referred to emphasized the need for better role-models than those provided by most television programmes and 'video nasties'. How to make the change? For the children of thoughtful parents who expose them to a variety of different influences the problem is less acute. It is otherwise with children in families disposed to violence who are likely to receive a strong reinforcing effect from what they watch nightly and are indoctrinated with the view that violence solves problems (Rutter, 1971, p. 240). Some improvement can be hoped for by helping parents to enrich their own lives. Basically, the problem demands long term interventions of many kinds in order to achieve even small changes.

Behaviour which might seem mindless and unintelligible to others makes sense once it is understood that children often fantasize about violent death as a way of escape from the stresses of family and school. Moreover, a most significant aspect of children's comments on their drawings is that delinquency and antisocial behaviour does not start at adolescence but is discernible at much earlier ages, even when no overt acts are committed.

MIDDLE-CLASS ANTISOCIAL BEHAVIOUR

Middle class crime committed by adults, especially embezzlement, does not receive much publicity unless it is on a large scale and newsworthy. On general grounds much of it is likely to be hidden or dealt with without recourse to the courts; it is present in forms hardly noticed by society. Children's behaviour is more uniform. In schools across the social spectrum they have to carry their belongings with them, otherwise they will disappear. The isolated boy with affluent parents who steals from his classmates is (like the working-class boy) sending out signals about needs not met just as much as his working-class peers. We do not know the extent of unhappiness in children from a middle-class background, but can surmise that a number suffer from unacknowledged emotional neglect which affects their behaviour. Expensive trendy clothes and super mountain bikes are not good substitutes.

APPROACHING ADOLESCENCE

As children approach adolescence, delinquent acts are likely to be a part of group behaviour, done without much thought when the opportunity presents itself. 'It's for a laugh,' they say, or 'we were bored, and anyway, everyone does it and I would be chicken if I didn't'. The problem can be related to the need to maintain a position in the group and gain peer approval rather than to psychological disturbance. But, although the reasons why some boys take risks which others resist should be addressed in terms of personality, this is not the full explanation: a social anthropologist's views on gang or group behaviour are equally relevant. In contrast, some teenagers adopt a criminal way of life as they attempt to find excitement or hide their lack of self-esteem: the criminal ambience will give them a place where they feel they belong.

PREVENTION

If the analysis suggested above is valid it is obvious that punishment for its own sake is irrelevant. What is more likely to change the pattern is intervention, starting with parenting skills in the very early years, followed by nursery education which has the primary aim of giving self-confidence. Schools need to provide a benign atmosphere where children can feel safe. In such schools many of these children have benefited from the care and concern of a sympathetic teacher. Those whose problems are deep-seated may respond to therapy which helps them to understand themselves and to change their image, or helps their families meet their needs more satisfactorily.

Some children displaying conduct disorders have managed reasonably well while young, but express their difficulties as teenagers and behave in a way which gives rise to more concern that the fairly general 'nuisance' behaviour of many adolescent boys in their search for a new identity and excitement. Usually girls of this age give a message of not feeling valued in different ways from boys but all may indicate distress by their destructive or antisocial behaviour.

To succeed, prevention must be extensive and long term, addressing relationships and the environment. Some positive preventive measures are listed below.

Parent Education

The National Children's Bureau has been concerned for a number of years with parent education and training, especially for those with preschool children. These and other schemes offer support and practical help in dealing with children's behaviour which is troublesome. Being consistent, not making threats or promises which are not carried out and remembering to comment and give encouragement for desired behaviour are among the techniques advocated, with positive results. Home Start, with 6000 voluntary workers also gives help and support with bringing up children.

The Child Development Programme, which is concerned to train Health Visitors, helps parents improve their skills and is successful because parents are encouraged to take control (Barker, 1994). In different areas a number of self-help parenting groups are also doing valuable work.

Family Centres

Family centres can play a very important part by providing experiences which help growth and development. They do this through groups where mothers discuss common problems and are encouraged to empathize with their children by talking to them and playing with them. A bonus for the mothers is that they gain confidence and make friends. If valuing the family has any meaning it is necessary to support and extend such community services.

Early Education

Long-term research in America found that those taught by High/ Scope principles at preschool level achieved higher educational results, particularly in reading skills, compared with a control group, and this remained so into adulthood.[8] More directly relevant to the present purpose, far fewer became delinquent. One technique used is to ask the children what activities they plan to do during the day. At the end of the session they report whether they have been successful.

Such a task is likely to give a message that activities can be planned in advance; important because one fairly general characteristic of delinquents is to react to a situation immediately without looking ahead. The delinquency-prevention effects were strongest among poor families. Programmes like these are effective probably because children learn that they have choices, and that they, their opinions and what they do, are of value. They learn to do things themselves. These important concepts help to reduce the negative effect of not having their needs met at home and affect their picture of themselves into adulthood.

Language, Speech and Reading

A number of studies have indicated that there may be a link between language and speech retardation which would identify some, though not all, antisocial behaviour at an early stage. Help with language development and reading are important preventive strategies.[9]

Multi-disciplinary Help

One other obvious remedy has been highlighted by a study conducted in the Isle of Wight (Rutter *et al.* 1970). A high proportion of children with psychiatric disorders were not receiving any help with their problems – a lack which emphasized the need for child and family clinics with a multi-disciplinary approach. Developing this service is especially important because the indications are that children who commit antisocial acts at an early age are likely to have more serious problems than those whose delinquent career starts in adolescence.

Family therapy can sometimes be effective by helping the family members relate to each other differently. The idea of 'children standing on an adult's shoulders' is useful in this context. If a child has a great deal of power or is holding his family or friends to ransom, it is worth considering if an adult is supporting him, whatever his behaviour. Vic was a real problem at school and in his neighbourhood because of his aggressive, destructive behaviour. He had no respect for any adult, never hesitating to respond to criticism with: 'My dad is a prize fighter. He'll soon come and sort you out.' In the end, all therapy failed and it was the law which sorted Vic out.

Conduct Disorder in the Social Context

It is unfortunate that some of the so-called help for children labelled delinquent, deviant or disturbed has strong political implications which take precedence over the needs of the child and ignore the findings of research, as, for example, the belief that the perpetrators need discipline or moral training. In the words of a former Home Secretary, Kenneth Clarke, they are 'nasty little juvenile offenders' – a view shared by Prime Minister John Major when he declared that society needs to 'condemn a little more and understand a little less'.[10] These views are not new, they were in operation in earlier decades in the form of approved schools and 'short, sharp shocks'. They did not diminish the amount of crime – if anything, the reverse – but 'tough on crime' is a very popular attitude and an understandable one if you have experienced a burglary, been mugged or had your car damaged. Anger, distress and a demand for punishment are normal reactions in the circumstances, but such feelings form a bad basis for law.

Linked with this view is the belief that the society and its institutions, especially the family, are responsible. Parents are too lax and fail to teach their children right from wrong; single parents or the increase in divorce are to blame, or schools are failing to discipline their charges. The solution is to introduce harsh regimes which emphasize discipline enforced by punishment. Too often it is punishing the victim.

A different approach is related to the reaction of society to the family. The implication is that there is one type of family comprising mum, dad and the kids, but this isn't the case now and never was, although in the past death was more likely to break up families than a failure in relationships. Forty per cent of children in Britain today have families whose income is less than half the average for the country and many of the children discussed above come from this group. Many live in substandard houses in the poor neighbourhoods of large cities. As previously said poverty is a factor because it makes the task of parenting more difficult and leads to people feeling alienated, depressed and angry.

Children also feel like this; as a friend of two ten-year old boys who had committed a very serious crime said 'They were just your average scruffs – like the rest of us'. But for the children and young people this could be countered in part by an imaginative youth service and leisure activities and by training schemes which realistically end in employment, if the problem was thought important.

More difficult is to make changes in family relationships because that involves changes in the status of women and in the value of mothering. The Children Act 1989 stresses the rights of children and the duties of parents. These need to be defined in terms of respect and warmth rather than control and punishment. Caring family relationships do not start at adolescence but are in evidence in the home life of younger children, hence the importance of high quality parenting and long-term preventive interventions, especially for the under-fives. It involves giving up the belief that all children come from happy homes and if they react to an unhappy environment, they should be punished.

Masculinity

Although it is very difficult to change any current belief in society, nevertheless, Yule's work on children's drawings quoted above suggests it is important to try. The conclusion from her analysis was that there should be a critical look at the destructive representations children are exposed to and counter the value put on 'whatever is fast, big, explosive, violent and expensive'. When assertion is confused with aggression, and macho identified with masculinity, can we wonder at the degree of violence shown by young boys? Finally, a comment made by a long-term prisoner at Risley Jail (BBC, 'Behind the Mask', January 1994): 'A man doesn't cry so the rage takes over – and this is where you end up.'

5 EMOTIONAL ABUSE AND PHYSICAL NEGLECT

EMOTIONAL ABUSE

One of the undoubted advances of the last half-century in understanding the less attractive aspects of society has been the recognition that some children are abused in their own home. Over the last thirty years a series of enquiries into distressing instances of brutality, and death in particular, have aroused public awareness: first of physical abuse, and then, more recently, of sexual abuse. But another form of abuse, one less often recognised, deserves discussion here.

Emotional abuse does not relate to one specific incident but to a sustained attack on a child's personality through belittling her abilities and development. It is differentiated from sexual abuse and physical abuse but often accompanies them; it can involve one child in the family or all of them. Because there are no tell-tale physical signs it is difficult to assess. Precisely because it is so common an attempt is made here to recognize its manifestations and understand its causes.

Essentially we are concerned with children whose parents, for many different reasons, have been unable to meet their needs appropriately, especially the first two needs discussed in this book – unconditional love, and respect for the child's personality. In innumerable ways parents' management is often unkind and damaging and can be incomprehensible to the child, who is not helped to develop as well as possible if treated in a way which undermines self-esteem. It may be that parents have failed to protect their child, not only from obvious danger but from repeated failure by expecting her to succeed at tasks which are patently beyond her. Other children are not protected from experiences unsuitable for their age. Some parents confuse the child because they react inappropriately, such as the mother who finds it amusing to see her child frightened or the father who, when his son fell down stairs, hit him for being clumsy. Others react with anger when they see their child sucking her thumb or using her body to comfort herself. The implication is not that it is wrong for parents to express anger; not to do so when a child knows that her behaviour is not acceptable will also cause confusion. What is undesirable is that anger expressed should attack the child's personality: You are always selfish/lazy/miserable/hopeless. Or it includes negative prophecies: you will end up in prison/on the streets/they'll take you away, and so on.

Most abused children have received some care but it has not been completely satisfactory. Maybe it was spasmodic or, after a good-enough start for the baby, warmth evaporated when the baby became a toddler.

The clues that all is not well may be quite small. Waiting in the checkout queue at the supermarket, a mother is trying very hard to engage her eighteen-month-old baby who is sitting in the trolley. She is talking rapidly to him, putting her face close to his, gesticulating and trying to get him to relate to her even when he turns his head away. The baby watches silently, unsmiling, detached. The mother perseveres; now moving the child's arms, now trying to get him to clap hands, but still there is no response. Then she tickles him and at last there is a reaction: he screams. In his distress he puts the button of his jacket in his mouth but his mother quickly removes it. He tries again and this time, annoyed, she snatches the jacket from him and throws it out of his reach into the trolley. He carries on screaming but his mother picks up a magazine, shutting him out. He might have been thought handicapped or autistic had he not previously responded to another child, showing clearly that neither was the case. No abuse as such, just two unhappy, frustrated people involved in an apparently trivial incident which might be indicative of a potentially worrying situation.

EARLY CHILDHOOD

Emotional abuse in infancy is correlated with non-organic failure to thrive. Sleep disturbance may be a pointer but the best indicator of abuse is shown by inadequate weight gain related to the act of feeding; persistently taking a long time, crying, falling asleep or vomiting while being fed may be indications of a baby's distress, symptoms which are especially worrying if the mother is depressed and cannot respond. The important skill a baby learns is to communicate her needs; if her messages are consistently ignored, or receive inappropriate responses, she could be handicapped in all areas of development.

Mrs Wilson thought her baby daughter, Tracy, did not like her because after her birth she did not smile as her mother had expected. In consequence Mrs Wilson did not talk to her and establish the close communication which would have encouraged such a response at around six weeks of age. She related to Tracy as if she were an adult who had disappointed her, and treated her without love; the baby was in serious danger of being neglected. Fortunately the situation changed when Mrs Wilson experienced mothering herself by the understanding staff of a Family Centre.

In nursery groups, such children often have difficulties because they have not learnt to trust. They relate to others by giving two messages: I want to play with you but I also want to hurt you – so the loving hug turns into a lethal squeeze. Their response to another child's distress is to add to it; just as they have not experienced sympathy themselves when distressed, so they are unable to empathize, identifying with the aggressor rather than with the hurt child. Further pointers indicating that there might be difficulties include a lack of spontaneity or even withdrawal. Poor concentration is a frequent symptom, while the failure to respond to comfort if hurt can indicate an unhappy child. Some try to solve their problems by being unusually dependent or unusually independent. All behaviour out of the ordinary needs to be thought about.

MIDDLE CHILDHOOD

An older child may also respond in these ways although, in the context of school, other signals indicate that the child might be experiencing emotional abuse at home. Teachers should be alert to children who are unwilling to mix with others or demonstrate aggressive spiteful behaviour. Some children learn from a very early age that being 'good', obedient and sitting still are acceptable, whilst expressing sadness, anxiety and asking for reassurance are not. If the experience of having feelings ignored or discounted is repeated often enough the child is put at a disadvantage in social situations. As with younger children, the ability to respond to others' feelings has not been learned because nobody has understood the child's distress; as a two-way process, communication is impaired.

Signs at school of unhappiness at home may include poor school attainment resulting from lack of concentration. Some of these children will be fantasizing about leaving home to find 'real' parents who care: some are greedy for the symbols of love like food and sweets; all have a lack of trust in adults that makes them difficult to help.

At home they play an important part in the family dynamics by taking all the 'badness' to themselves, allowing other family members to be regarded as 'good'. Some never give up hope of being loved and constantly try to please, becoming the Cinderellas of the family. They cannot talk about their unhappiness because they feel they must protect either their siblings or parents. Sadly, unexpressed resentment, paranoia or helplessness often masks their true feelings and does not always arouse the sympathy of other people; their role of victim has been well learned. Their overwhelming need for closeness can have the opposite effect on teachers who are not tuned to their distress.

Emotional abuse has many manifestations. 'Abuse' may seem too strong a word for some of these situations compared with that of children who suffer physical violence or sexual abuse, but the effects can be just as devastating and the harm done can last for years.

Verbal abuse can lead to unpleasant consequences for children. Some are obsessed with wanting to hurt themselves or someone else; fear of being hurt by other people or of external events may dominate their lives. Some years ago, Ney (1986) conducted a study of fifty-seven American children, and found that those exposed to verbal abuse were likely to believe that there would be a nuclear war and that they would be killed in it, a striking demonstration of the lack of hope many of these children feel.

NEGLECT OF EMOTIONAL NEEDS

By this is meant the failure to carry out the parental tasks in a way expected in a particular culture. It embraces talking and listening to children, playing with them, providing stimulation and expressing pleasure in their achievements as well as keeping the child safe; all time-consuming but necessary demonstrations of valuing and respecting the child. Failure in these areas will not necessarily be disastrous or fatal to development but are a sign of inadequate child care. The reasons for this failure by parents are likely to be related to their own lack of good experience as children, poor health or high stress levels or an unawareness that these shared activities are important for development. Parents who see their children as burdens will refuse their attempts at closeness, giving them no experience of being wanted, let alone enjoyed; shared pleasure of achievements will be non-existent. The teacher of a five-year-old who was treated in this way discovered he did not know that he had a birthday like other children.

Jonathan's academic parents were caring but had no idea how to meet his needs, except by intellectual stimulation. At four he could describe the plumbing system in his house but in his play group he was quite unable to relate to other children or engage in pretend play. In no way could he be said to be abused in the sense of being harmed, but he had not been given any help in developing his emotional and social abilities, or provided with the necessary tools for communicating with other children. In such a situation there is the danger that the initial problem may be compounded by later frustrations caused by feeling isolated or different.

The complex factors contributing to a child's being emotionally neglected can relate to the parents' relationships past and present, the child's personality and appearance, or the family's environment. Sometimes children with a step-parent or those with a different parent from the other children may be in this category, or the child's personality may not 'fit' the parents': for example, the quiet child in a boisterous family or the physically less capable child in a family of athletes. Other patterns which lead to an unsatisfactory child-parent relationship are outlined below (Chapter 8); parental guilt about the neglect and anger at not feeling good about their child are usually present.

Casual remarks can carry unexpected weight. A nurse, saying to the mother of a new baby who is having difficulty in sucking, 'You've got a right one here, I've never known such a wilful baby', can unintentionally label an infant in a negative way at a time when the mother is most susceptible. Such comments, forgotten by most mothers, but impressing deeply those unsure of themselves in their new role, can lead to babies being rejected.

If the mother does not develop close protective feelings and there is no rapport between her and her baby, the baby is likely to be miserable, its crying making the mother feel first despair, then anger. Small signs of this happening could be the mother's lack of eye contact, or avoidance of touch, or holding the baby at the end of her lap rather than closely. Or the baby will be fed with the bottle propped up on a cushion, the mother explaining that she doesn't like to be held and is happier this way. The baby's perception can be inferred to be quite different. She has given messages about wanting to play or being hungry and uncomfortable but no one heard. Crying relieves the tension but the belief that this is a hostile world, a world which can't understand signals, persists. Safer, then, to accept not being held and to withdraw in an attempt to survive the despair and confusion.

From about five years old those who are rejected will have the same sort of feelings, although they are not correlated so directly with bodily needs. At times their anger will be kept inside, stored until it can be given expression against somebody or something else or directed against themselves. Children in this situation cannot be straightforwardly angry; feelings of compassion for unfeeling parents further confuses their thoughts.

Children with a different kind of personality will openly express the anger arising from the situation accompanied by the belief that people are unreliable and hostile. One way in which the rejected child survives is by being ready to attack, but, despite overwhelming odds, rejected children are usually loath to give up the hope that one day a miracle will happen and they will be loved, a hope that will cause some unconsciously to resist growing up.

One effect can be a feeling that, if nobody loves them, no one feels sad or concerned if they get into trouble. As they have not let anyone down there is little shame or regret. Change comes when they learn that they do not deserve this sort of treatment – it is what has happened to them which is bad, not themselves.

What follows is a discussion of some principal types of abuse which parents may unwittingly commit and teachers, social workers and others in the helping professions need to recognise. The list is not exhaustive.

OSTRACIZED CHILDREN

Certain characteristics are shared by children who are consistently ignored by their family. As babies they are left to cry in a bedroom or to sit in baby-chairs for hours on end and given only very spasmodic stimulation. They are likely to be backward in speech because nobody speaks to them, and their intelligence is often impaired because they have not been encouraged to explore, to experiment, to learn by playing, to be curious and to think through problems. 'What would happen if ...?', is not a question these deprived children have learned to ask. Many seem lethargic and passive, appearing good to the casual onlooker.

For these children the experience of being ignored can continue at school unless they are lucky enough to find a teacher who will enhance their self-esteem. For others less fortunate the pattern is reinforced: if they do not present behaviour problems and attract attention, or are disruptive, they go unnoticed. Sadly, unless they are understood, they are not among the more rewarding pupils because of their poor social skills; they carry the extra burden of an all-pervading stressful internal world which makes it hard for them to concentrate, to trust, to take risks. Difficulty in committing things to paper and in understanding symbols makes number work especially hard and can indicate a child under stress. They are unable to use their potential to learn. What ignored children learn about themselves has far-reaching consequences for them emotionally and educationally.

Similarly, those who are excluded from family activities suffer a great deal. Richard, aged seven, a doctor's son, was made to stay in an attic throughout the weekend as a punishment. His daydreams were of all sorts of terrible tortures which he would inflict on 'his enemies', each one worse that the last. Rod, also seven, who had a different father to his siblings, was never allowed to have his meals with the family, even on Christmas Day. In order to survive he retreated into a fantasy world more vivid to him than life. One day his real father who was very rich would take him away and buy him a super bike and given him as much food as he could eat and really, really love him. Not surprisingly, at school both Richard and Rod were labelled 'dreamers'.

Some excluded children are denied family pleasures on the grounds that 'We can't take him with us, he would play up and spoil it for everyone else', and are also denied money for school trips and other events because they don't deserve treats. Observant teachers are aware of a child treated differently from other children in the family.

Parents who sulk need to be mentioned here. They surround themselves with a wall of silence that the child cannot penetrate. This can be a punishment worse than some physical abuse – a cold, calculated rejection which carries with it a statement about parents being all-powerful while at the same time the desperate child may not know what she has done wrong and certainly has no idea when her ordeal will end. Even when it is over she knows no peace of mind. It can so easily happen again because of her wickedness. She thinks that if she has caused a parent to feel so much anger that it cannot be given expression in words, then she must be a very bad child indeed.

TEASED CHILDREN

A second group of emotionally abused children are those ridiculed and laughed at and subjected to constant teasing – activities normally felt by adults to be quite harmless. What is really happening is that they are being used in a subtle, aggressive way, belittled and confused for adults' pleasure and enjoyment. Unfortunately, many parents, fathers especially, who relate to their children in this way justify themselves by saying 'He's got to learn to take a joke'. The same response may be given to a child upset by sarcasm.

Seven-year-old Kim, a tense little girl who had never enjoyed food, provides an example of inappropriate parental handling undermining self-esteem. Because she did not eat her dinner her parents teased her by saying she would have only cabbage to eat for a whole week. She began to feel distressed but her parents were unaware of this. With eyes filled with tears she said 'Why do you keep teasing me?'. The parents laughed and the mother replied: 'Because we enjoy it, and when you are a mother with a little girl you will be able to tease her'. 'I'll never, I'll never', cried Kim, and to the sound of her parents' laughter she ran upstairs to cry on her bed. Such thoughtlessness was completely atypical for these parents, who were kindness itself to other people but used their daughter to express unacknowledged feelings relating to their own powerlessness as children.

Other parents excel at the 'double bind' technique. 'Come here and give me a kiss', says the father. When the little boy approaches his father he is told: 'Go away, you're a poof'. Repeated experiences of this kind convince the child that he can never win. He does not know whether he is loved and does not understand that he is being used by his father who, while feeling powerful and dominant, is freed from the guilt he would feel if the child were being physically abused.

CRITICIZED CHILDREN

Children who are constantly criticized can also be regarded as emotionally abused. Even a small baby who does not understand the words will pick up negative feelings by the tone of voice. A timid child frightened of fights, or who is not athletic, may have a hard time if his father wants a macho son. Obviously not all children with such insensitive parents can be called emotionally abused, and only if criticism is the usual way of communicating with the child is this the correct phrase. Children who are constantly deprecated by their parents can become the scapegoats for all the family; then their isolation and loneliness is complete. If this is how they are treated at home, and possibly at school, too, they feel as children do in so many situations, that they must be to blame.

CHILDHOOD DENIED: BOUNDARIES CROSSED

Emotional deprivation takes innumerable forms, but frequently the children are used to meet the emotional needs of parents. Mandy's mother, with her pigtails and little white socks, needed her six-year-old daughter as a companion; someone on whom she could be emotionally dependent. Mandy was not allowed to visit friends or to go on school trips and had to come home straight from school because her mother needed her too much to let her develop independently. Any tentative friendships the child made had been quickly discouraged when she started school. Superficially, it looked as if she had given up her wish to mix with other children because she felt safer with Mummy, but in reality there was a conflict, her infantilism not being what she really wanted. She expressed her anger indirectly by biting holes in the sleeves of her sweaters.

A different group comprises those children who are acting like parents to their parents. This can happen when the parents, because of their own experiences as children, crave for a close relationship, but at the same time are unable to trust anyone to achieve this. They may marry an equally inadequate partner, then, unaware that successful parenting is first about giving, not taking, fantasize that the child will give them the loving relationship which has eluded them.

In this situation the children have to protect their parents, comforting them and taking inappropriate responsibility. In a sense, they are powerful but are also abused because they fail to do what the parent unconsciously expects of them. They are not helped to surmount the development hurdles and all their emotional energy goes into meeting the needs of their child-parent. As a child with this background said, 'I am nobody', meaning he was only there to meet his parent's needs – his own didn't count and therefore he didn't count.

This pattern may occur, understandably, in some lone parent families where the human need for comfort is obvious. Michelle had become the 'parent' in her family because, following a bereavement, her mother became depressed and for a time was incapable of caring for her younger children. Unfortunately, once the pattern was established she became her mother's comforter and confidante. She enjoyed the advantages of this situation but over time came to resent the responsibility, her anger erupting in an atypical attack on a girl at school. Luckily, her school appreciated that it was a 'cry for help' and meetings with mother and daughter helped them to change the pattern.

If parents have to deny the feelings of the child, she, in consequence, becomes even more confused. 'You worry about me, don't you dear?'. For the child this is a burden; it is not safe to be openly angry and any opposition is interpreted by the parent as rejection. Family meetings expose this kind of relationship and can help to free the child of such responsibility.

Sometimes the mutual dependence between inadequate parents is so strong as to arouse their anger, because nobody wants to be completely powerless. A child can receive this anger because of the impossibility of her being able to meet all the needs of her immature parents.

Emotional abuse can be more subtle. For example, when a parent's life is ruled by his or her need to have a precocious child, the encouragement given can appear benign. That is not so at all if the child's emotional and social needs are sacrificed in the pursuit of parental ambition, because the child is burdened with concepts of success and failure at an early age. She will wish to please these good parents who have made such sacrifices on her behalf, but hand in hand with the wish for success can be an intense anxiety and guilt about the possibility of failing to come up to expectations.

A particularly difficult situation occurs when the child takes over the care of a physically ill parent. When, as it usually is, the caring is done with love, it is quite wrong to call it abuse, yet if the effect of too much responsibility is to stunt the child's normal emotional development it can be damaging. Obviously, relatives, friends and community services can help a great deal to share the responsibility, but for an adolescent in such circumstances it can be particularly difficult to incorporate feelings of love into the normal teenage desire for independence. Such children are often lonely and in need of an understanding relative or friend to talk to, while others welcome the help of a skilled counsellor or someone who can answer their questions. The need to care causes some to miss school and a few are embarrassed by their situation.

This is not emotional abuse in the usual sense, especially as many children are pleased to help and gain in confidence by doing so, but, nevertheless, there can be a great burden of responsibility for a child, on top of the normal stresses of child-parent relationships: the fear of the parent being put in an institution or of having to go into care themselves if they can't manage, may be a hidden thought – a chasm to avoid falling into at all costs.

CHILDREN WHO LACK CONTINUITY

A group of parents has been identified under the label 'chaotic' (Trowell and Castle, 1981). They were characterized by their lack of organization and motivation for change and were often in conflict with authority; their behaviour and relationships with their children were difficult to alter in any way. Such personalities will not be able to meet their children's needs for continuity and security and although, again, 'abuse' may be too strong a word, the degree of harm done depends upon the children's personalities and other influences they experience.

Another definable group is that of mothers who have volatile, mercurial personalities, full of energy at times but also subject to bouts of depression. Mothers with this psychological make-up will find parenthood especially difficult if they are not supported by other adults, or when there are extra stresses such as illness or marital problems. They are able to respond consistently neither to the child's distress nor her pleasure, because their own inner emptiness is too great. In time the child gives up hope of being able to rely on uniform responses and becomes confused by what is experienced at times as the withdrawal of love. Similar effects are observable in a child whose mother is an alcoholic. It is as if she has two mothers. Confusion, self-doubt, guilt and anger can become an emotionally-draining, hidden part of her mental life.

CHILDREN LEFT ALONE

Some mothers who, for whatever reason, need to go to work leave their preschool children alone in the house, sometimes for many hours. Others have to play outside, unsupervised. Often the mothers are not deliberately neglectful and feel guilty but cannot find a better solution; childcare provisions are too expensive or non-existent. It is a significant problem; for example, one London police district deals each month with about twenty-seven children left unsupervised (Channel 4, December 1993).

Although it is natural to feel sympathy for the plight of these mothers, they are, in fact, solving their problem in a way which fails to meet their child's emotional needs. Children must have the mutual caring exchanges which are vital for good development. Lack of stimulation and an unsatisfied curiosity may well affect their intellectual development; their fears relating to long isolation go unheeded. This is yet another instance where the child's needs are not given priority. Some will use their own bodies for comfort or to express their anger; many will become lethargic and depressed when their unheard cries of protest and despair echo around an empty house.

We cannot condone a solution which is likely to cause emotional harm to a child. The financial or child-care arrangements made by the Government are not of concern here, but society certainly needs to address the problem with some urgency.

SERIOUSLY EMOTIONALLY-DEPRIVED CHILDREN

The very small proportion of children who have experienced little or no emotional warmth present far more serious problems and need long-term specialist help. They may be diagnosed as suffering from childhood psychoses (sometimes incorrectly), are deeply damaged and need psychiatric help and are outside the scope of this book.

PHYSICALLY NEGLECTED CHILDREN

It is difficult to decide which of the principal categories of abuse physical neglect has most affinity with, but since it often arises by default, resulting from parents' own mental states rather than deliberate cruelty, the matter is as appropriate here as anywhere. If children are not kept safe or are exposed to repeated danger, their anxieties increase. If parents fail to set limits appropriate for the child's age and culture by, for instance, allowing the child to be destructive of others' property, their non-intervention is taken to imply approval.

Neglect can occur when parents do not provide adequate food, clothing and supervision or maintain acceptable standards of cleanliness; some may not allow their children freedom to leave the home for leisure or recreation, thus making them virtual prisoners. The children are likely to be in poorer health than others and failure to seek medical attention when necessary may be another sign of neglect. Parents' low intelligence, mental illness or their own childhood history of abuse and neglect can contribute to the problem; some are drug- or alcohol-abusers and a few have aggressive, sadistic personalities. It is likely that a number of such parents are suffering from unacknowledged depression; it is this which leads to their hopelessness and thus their inability to make the necessary changes in child-rearing.

The effect of physical neglect on the child's emotional health cannot be underestimated, for all that the latter is a by-product of the former. To give just one apparently trivial example: a child being sent to school in the depths of winter in a thin summer dress experiences discomfort and, in addition, her self-esteem is undermined because she feels different from the other children. Other neglected children have not had their physical ailments attended to: for example, ear infections in two- and three-year-olds, if untreated can affect language development.

Families where children are neglected can be isolated and alienated from others. They may feel that those trying to help have a hidden agenda which is alien to their needs and wishes, a belief which causes them to misinterpret the benign actions of others. They may also see things as black or white; if people – or services – are not perfect, then they are useless. Some are suspicious of those in authority and resist intervention from outside. Families like these might respond to a trusted health visitor or care worker giving practical help, such as assisting with the children, ensuring appointments are kept, and so on. Weekend respite care may be enough to make the difference between managing or the child being fostered. Family Centres and other services which give parents companionship and support, and teach parenting skills in a way which is enjoyable and acceptable, provide a valuable preventative service. There is a great deal which needs to be done.

DISCUSSION OF EMOTIONAL ABUSE AND PHYSICAL NEGLECT

What constitutes emotional abuse changes as knowledge about mental and physical health advances. Twenty years ago, we did not know that it was harmful for pregnant mothers to smoke. Does this mean that mothers who ignore such advice today are negligent by putting their baby at risk, or should this be a matter for personal choice? Should a parent be allowed to tease a child or make him eat meals away from the family without interference? It is inconceivable that the law should ever intervene in these close personal situations but, nevertheless, parents should be aware of the damage they can do. We can't use a government health warning, like that on a cigarette packet, but a way needs to be found to help parents do their best for their children.

What degree of threat is tantamount to emotional abuse today? It was acceptable in the nineteenth century to control children by fear of damnation, hell or divine punishment. More recently, children were threatened that the policeman would take them away if they were naughty, or 'I'll put you in a Home'. 'If you are naughty. Mummy will leave you and never, never come back', is a powerful modern-day equivalent. All these threats can do emotional damage to a child, threatening fundamental security because a small child is very reluctant to question seriously what adults do and say. They are harmful to some degree, but do they amount to emotional abuse? Where should we draw the line? How far should we be concerned to intervene when actions lead to emotional damage to the child? At present we value the rights of the individual very highly while the checks provided by a closely-knit community are not so general in these days of isolated families.

There are many pitfalls in intervention. If the family's way of relating to one another is aggressive, its members communicating by shouting, threatening or perpetual 'put-down' comments, the effect on children varies, those with robust personalities being less affected than timid sensitive ones. In families where such communication can be distressing for the outsider to hear, and even if we believe that the children will repeat the pattern, we are not justified in taking action unless there is clear evidence that a child is suffering. Not a few children find ways of meeting their needs for warmth and encouragement and for being valued, from caring adults outside the family or, as they grow older, supportive peer groups.

We also have to be careful to respect the child-rearing methods of black families and other ethnic groups – white middle-class people do not have a monopoly on good childcare practice.

Neglected children pose a problem for social workers. In families where relationships are warm and caring but the children are ill-fed and do not experience 'good-enough' parenting, despite encouraging the parents to meet their children's needs, should the children be moved? Parents resent this not only because of the heart-break but because, often rightly, they feel that if they were given the allowance a foster mother receives then their children would not be neglected. Poverty leads to depression which leads to inadequate parenting. Some parents, of course, would neglect their children however much money they received because of their own damaged personalities and inability to appreciate what is required to avoid having unhappy children. Nevertheless, quite a high proportion of neglected children come from families burdened by the interrelated practical and emotional consequences of poverty. Unless the numbers of unemployed are reduced and the issue of second families is addressed with sensitivity the numbers will increase.

Other kinds of emotional abuse might seem less important in the light of some of the neglected children's suffering but, nevertheless, all abuse is potentially harmful. While physical neglect is a criminal offence, as yet there are no accepted criteria for compulsory intervention in the other situations described above. If, as is being increasingly realized, the consequences of psychological maltreatment are detrimental to a child's emotional and physical development, then some strategies should be devised to deal with the problem, including training for parenthood, especially for boys.

Nowadays we have some idea of why parents abuse. Some of the causes can be changed more easily than others; some relate to personality and relationships while other are more fundamental to society in general. We have much to learn about ways in which to approach the whole problem, but what is certain is that any serious attempt to improve the care of children overall would need finer assessment techniques and multiple approaches in the long term. It would require early intervention which addresses distorted parent-child relationships, probably involving the whole family.

This is a difficult area because of the problem of finding a control group, but it is important to know in what circumstances fostering is a better alternative to the child's home. We need to be able to evaluate a number of different aspects of the family – the quality of the parental relationship, what resources are available, the emotional climate, impulse control, the power structure, communication, and how much family members respect each other, as well as listening to their suggestions about what they think would be best and what changes could be made, because the situation is one which has to be altered.

Some of the situations that children experience are discussed above; what is beyond doubt to those involved professionally is that far too many are unhappy. Dr Kellmer Pringle (1975), when discussing the child's need for love and security, wrote that this need is met 'by the child experiencing from birth onwards a continuous, reliable, loving relationship'. Giving encouragement and creating circumstances where this kind of relationship can thrive should take precedence over everything else.

6 PHYSICAL AND SEXUAL ABUSE

Much has been written about physical and sexual abuse. As this book is concerned with the feelings of children it focuses on the emotional impact on a child and the long term consequences; the feelings of parents are also discussed, though not the psychology of abuse in depth. Neither diagnostic interviewing nor the procedures and legal matters are included. Suffice to say that the immediate response to the discovery of abuse must be to keep the child safe and to end the violence.

PHYSICAL ABUSE

THE CHILDREN

It is more than thirty years since the phrase 'battered baby syndrome' was used and physical abuse, or NAI (Non-Accidental Injury), became a matter of general concern. It is a difficult subject to talk to children about because one effect of abuse is to inject a degree of fear or lack of trust into all relationships; consequently children believe, all too often, that adults will accept other adults' view that they were naughty and therefore to blame. A further dimension to the problem is that many want to protect their parents, whose goodness and love they believe in, whatever happens. With any type of abuse, what also has to be kept in mind is that even if events appear very similar, each child will experience them in a unique way.

Physically abused children may be surprisingly young. Half of those in an NSPCC sample (Dale, 1986) were under twelve months old, and a few years earlier at the Park Hospital a study found that two thirds were in this age group. Such young children do not have the ability to express themselves in words, thereby adding to frustration on both sides. It is not surprising that babies under two years old appear more likely to be severely abused than older children.

The literature on the subject tends to assume that children are abused by their parents, but probably many are abused by older siblings or step-siblings, especially those close in age and girls with aggressive brothers. Parents sometimes condone this behaviour, believing that this is to be expected and 'boys will be boys'.

WAYS IN WHICH ABUSED CHILDREN SURVIVE

An abused child has to develop ways of emotional survival; one of them is denial. Six-year-old Gary, an only child, needed his father's love so much that he accepted the physical pain of the beatings he received, believing he deserved such punishment. His stoicism helped him to accept the very painful treatment he need for a physical condition, but he insisted that his father took him whenever he had to go to hospital. This was the only time he received paternal praise. Without help in understanding his feelings, Gary could become an aggressive parent himself, identifying with his strong father and covering up feelings of low esteem by aggressive acts.

Some children learn to detach themselves from the abuse. One instance is Buster Keaton, a film comedian well-known in the 1920s and 1930s, who was part of his parents' theatrical act as a very young child (Miller, 1990). However much they abused him on stage he had to show no reaction to the pain. This experience left him, as an adult, with the inability to show any emotion, even to smile. To be completely submissive may help avoid physical damage; unfortunately it cannot protect against psychological damage. Detachment, then, is one way to survive. Other children who desperately love their abusing parent are grateful because at least they are not ignored and believe they must have asked for the punishment.

At the time of abuse fear prevents an aggressive reaction being expressed. Boys are inclined to store up their feelings until they are stronger or may bully younger children, although some adopt the role of victim throughout life. Girls are especially likely to direct their anger inwards or to become excessively anxious. Obviously, there are many exceptions to this observation, as is apparent in the number of abused girls who, in their attempt to deal with feelings associated with the pain they experienced as a child, grow up to become difficult adolescents or aggressive women. Those who cling to the role of victim expect to be treated badly, unconsciously making decisions which cause the pattern to be repeated.

Whatever the later manifestations, physically abused children are likely to have a poor self-image and lack confidence. Such distressing experiences will divert emotional energy towards dealing with the fear and anger evoked by the event, rather than directing it in the normal channel towards growing and learning. It is not surprising that they are less healthy than their peers and less able to concentrate. Despite what has happened, or is happening, young abused children accept the parents they have. A few might want to leave home, but for the majority this is the situation they know and understand, and amid the violence and pain they do have a place; to send them away is often experienced as a punishment, depriving them of their identity. The need to belong is strong. Generally, it is only later that abused children leave their parents; abused adolescents form part of the army of homeless young people who sleep in the streets today.

A great deal has been written about identifying abused children, mostly by observing carefully their appearance and demeanour and noting bodily signs such as bruising, burns, broken bones, weals, bites, scalding and other injuries. Besides these observable external clues there are two less obvious and contrasting symptoms of abuse: what has been called 'frozen watchfulness', and the inability to keep still. Gary, discussed above, was a particularly striking example of the first: through half-closed eyes he observed his father's every move, his body remaining tense and immobile. At the opposite extreme are those who attempt to hide their anxiety behind bright chatter; over-friendly without discrimination. Young babies often have a distinctive, quiet high-pitched cry which indicates a fear of being noticed and a hopelessness about being comforted.

In families where a child is physically abused there may be some correlation with a failure to bond, isolation, or stress in the home, but this is not always so. Many families struggling against insuperable odds do not inflict injury on their children, although it does seem probable that parents who physically hurt their children have experienced hurt when they were growing up. We know less about those who do not repeat the pattern.

LONG TERM EFFECTS

Parents in Victorian England and earlier saw it as a duty to chastise their children in order to inculcate obedience and to break the child's will, but patterns varied in different periods of history and in different social classes. According to one eminent historian, 'most children in history have not been loved or hated, or both, by their parents, they have been neglected or ignored' (Stone, 1981).

Possibly, in the light of this remark, the high historic death rate among children was related to emotional as well as physical factors.

Today, physically abused children, especially those who have been shaken violently, can suffer some degree of brain damage leading to mental handicap; language delay can also be a consequence, especially if the accompanying degree of emotional neglect or abuse is great. Many more will be socially handicapped because of their lack of self-esteem and overriding fear.

As adults, familiar with violence as a way of life, they may unconsciously seek a partner who has had the same experience or at least will go along with it. Too often these children grow up not wanting to perpetuate the pattern but the spectre of violence is waiting to emerge in the next generation when their own child is being difficult or demanding. When child victims become adults the violence can be a life sentence requiring great control to keep the potential aggressive behaviour contained and controlled. The cost in mental energy is high, the self-hate at times unbearable.

THE PARENTS

In an attempt to hide even from themselves the lack of warmth for their infant or their fear of losing control, parents may be excessively tidy and the baby beautifully clothed. Not trusting others, they keep their true feelings hidden from inquisitive authorities, even if they are desperate for help and live in fear that one day they will cause a tragedy. These unspoken appeals need to be picked up and acted upon by professional workers.

In many different ways, a child reactivates in the parent unresolved problems from the past, especially the feeling of not being cherished, which is something the baby cannot do; it is the baby who needs cherishing. Parents report that they cannot stand the crying; they do not want to abuse but when tiredness is added to the feelings of failure they become angry and hit their baby who, by her tears, was merely asking for comfort. The tears can be, for the parent, a reminder of their own unexpressed sadness, for abusing parents have had sad lives, marred by the loss of a happy childhood. The pattern can change if parents are helped to become more in touch with their own helplessness and unacknowledged resentment arising from the fact that, as children, they were not comforted. These are the feelings which inhibit empathy for their own child.

For others, food is emotive; because of their own deprivation and lack of nurture in the past they still need to receive. The baby's cry of hunger can feel like an intolerable sign of greed. Caring for a new baby, of which feeding plays a large part, is primarily about giving by responding to the baby's demands.

Some deprived mothers experience their babies only in relation to themselves: he cries to spite me; She's crying in order to punish me for being a bad mum; Because I wasn't well she made herself sick; He's so greedy, he's wanting food all the time, he's got to learn to wait; She doesn't love me, therefore I can't love her. These babies who are not having their needs met are experienced by their own mothers as persecuting parents, and in consequence they are at risk.

For one mother, her small son was like her aggressive husband. The punches she gave her baby were those she was too frightened to give her husband who hit her as her father had done. She was unwittingly contributing towards perpetuating an undesirable situation until she could perceive the baby as a person in his own right who needed the loving care that only she could give him.

Vicarious violence can take a different form. When reports of deliberately injured children appear in the press the question often asked is why the non-abusing parent didn't stop it. Sometimes a battered wife fails to act because she is obsessed by the husband and feels grateful that he has, so far, saved her life. More often she is just too frightened. Only very occasionally does a mother in these circumstances enjoy seeing a frightened child or the father-figure being violent. This is a pleasure manifested by the few mothers who collude in their partners' battering of their children, sometimes to death. When, probably much later, the child realises that her mother could have protected her but failed to do so, desolation knows no bounds. No longer can she think that at least Mummy loved her; the child's growing awareness that neither parent cared is heart-breaking to watch.

The need to be loved is so powerful that the anger at being deprived, unwanted or unvalued cannot be expressed directly. It is common to find adults maintaining that the punishment they received as a child was deserved, citing incidents which could be interpreted as love. Dad gave me his old penknife. Once he took me to the fair. Anything to preserve the myth that this was a good parent who did love his child.

Denial notwithstanding, the anger must be expressed somewhere and when there is a small, helpless child and plenty of reasons for 'punishment', there is a risk of history repeating itself.

Original sin is no longer in fashion. Instead: the child needs discipline; she has to learn who is boss here; it's for her own good; I can't stand a spoilt child; it's a harsh world, and she has to be prepared for it; and – the most frequent and thoughtless comment – I was hit as a child and it didn't do me any harm. The truth of this is difficult to ascertain and such a negative approach is not a good basis for child-rearing. This kind of thinking, which is widespread, finds some sympathy among those who are concerned to help, without their approval of punitive behaviour which goes 'too far'. It is a fallacy. These are parents who see violence as an integral part of parenting and are fearful of losing control over many things, including the child. They want 'respect' from the child even if it is based on fear. Their needs are paramount, not the child's.

Sometimes the abuse stems from an uncharacteristic loss of control because some external factor – the father's redundancy, for example – is causing the parent anger or anxiety. It will be followed by remorse and distress, but is worrying because once a parent has hit a child it is easier to repeat the abuse. Some children have a parent who is loving much of the time but becomes violent under the influence of drink; the next day they may deny with complete conviction that the bruisings and breakages were anything to do with them, leaving the children hurt and confused.

Abuse may stem from a further, and, to many, improbable cause: the lack, on the part of the parents of any realistic expectation of age-appropriate behaviour. Susan, aged eighteen months, was expected to eat with a knife and fork and her crying, when she was upset, brought an angry response. Neighbours reported her screams when she was hit with a wooden spoon for wetting the bed. Subsequently, a health visitor helped her mother to meet Susan's needs in an appropriate way.

Some children have to care for the younger children in the family. Five-year-old Phil was often beaten for failing to care for his small brother adequately. His plight was only known to the authorities because he scalded himself while preparing his baby brother's bottle and had to be taken to hospital where his bruises and healed fractures were noticed. Because of impossible expectations these children are likely to grow up expecting failure. What they do is not valued, what they fail to do is punishable.

Some emotionally impoverished parents who expect the child to love them can interpret the look of a very young baby as a rejection. Mrs Jones thought her baby looked at her in a hostile way while being fed. She threw her across the room, thinking that if the baby hated her then she hated the baby. She saw herself as a bad person and expected to have a bad child, therefore the imagined hostility confirmed her belief and affected the relationship with her daughter for many years.

Having too many children close together may make for depressed and overburdened parents who lack the emotional energy to meet all the family's needs, especially if they are poor or live in overcrowded conditions. Even so, those who have lifelines in the form of helpful friends and relations, and are able to use what assistance the state provides, will manage.

Parents who abuse their children come from any social background, but the overburdened and underprivileged families, because they are more likely to be known to the authorities, are more easily identified. Inadequate personalities with a low threshold of tolerance, or with experience of physical violence in their childhood at home or at school, may be found at any level of society.

DIFFICULT-TO-HELP PARENTS

A few children are part of the delusional system of their psychotic parents. Some have parents with sadistic personalities who torture them; others have parents with serious alcohol or drug problems. Sometimes it is necessary for the children to be removed from home in the hope of their making affectionate bonds with other caring adults, and occasionally, when the relationship is too destructive, the bonds between abusing parent and child have to be severed. Often these are inadequate, unstable parents who interpret the actions of others as persecutory; when in a state of fear they are liable to attack, and at such times children are especially vulnerable. Counselling, family therapy, shared care (where the child is placed in a weekly residential educational establishment) and therapeutic work with families, by the NSPCC for example, are successful in keeping some of them with their parents, but the needs of the children have to come first.

Serious injury to children is usually, though not always, caused by men who believe masculinity is about being hard and strong; feelings of tenderness have to be denied. For this pattern to change there will have to be an acceptance that good parenting is not instinctive but is learnt from being exposed to a different approach to children, one which is concerned to understand their needs and increase their self-esteem.

WHAT HELPS ABUSED AND NEGLECTED CHILDREN?

A first step would be universal acknowledgement that all abuse and neglect is harmful and must be followed by action. To blame parents is often not the best way, for they are victims of their upbringing and all too often they are troubled or under pressure and lack adequate resources or the necessary knowledge. Some have personalities too damaged to meet their child's needs, but the majority do what they can with limited personal and material resources.

Preventive work, with boys as well as girls, includes discussions at school concerning family relationships and responsibilities. The message must be that having a baby is not just having a baby but taking responsibility for the emotional and physical development of a child for many years and is therefore a very long commitment which requires different skills. Education for parenthood which suggests that children can be brought up without violence and fear, but with concern and co-operation, can be a revelation. There is much to be done before a baby is born.

Also necessary are empathy and knowledge about what behaviour can be expected at different ages. Equally important is an understanding that a crying baby is not deliberately provoking but is giving a message about something missing, a difficult concept for those whose own needs for care were not met. Some have to learn to accept the baby they have, not the one they imagined. The baby is neither a rejecting parent, nor their demanding spouse, nor their unhappy, unsatisfied self. Neither is it a pseudo-parent destined to give emotional support rather than to receive it.

The contribution of post-natal depression to neglect or abuse is still not as fully appreciated as it should be, especially if there are difficulties and the mother leaves hospital before the baby. Often, too, abusing parents are physically unwell, suffering from a number of minor ailments which need to be dealt with. It is harder to be patient if something hurts.

Some sensitive social services departments and voluntary bodies contribute by providing, among other things, shared care, family aides and family centres. Home Start helps a great many families, and health visitors are often described as a lifeline by over-burdened mothers. The benefits of good day nurseries and skilled childminders are well known. Residential placements for the whole family in order to establish bonding and improve parental skills is another valuable service for a few. Self-help groups, 'drop-in' centres and training in social skills all help to alleviate loneliness and improve skills in parenting and in managing anger. They are far more likely to be successful if parents feel they have some control over the interventions.

Therapy concerned with improving communication and showing warmth to children can be helpful. There are examples of a few schemes which teach parents to appreciate and respond to their child's needs by shared play. Parents learn to use clear communication to share the enjoyment of the activities. The technique involves giving undivided attention and conveying pleasure for approved behaviour while ignoring most of the unacceptable behaviour. This approach needs to be extended. The benefits are likely to be an improvement in parental skills, and thus their self-esteem, to the benefit of the child. Abused children might also need individual therapy to help them come to terms with their ambivalent feelings and to learn to have confidence in themselves.

Finally, resources channelled into reducing the problems of all kinds of abuse and neglect at the earliest opportunity could not fail to be beneficial. What is not helpful is for any social workers involved to be blamed almost automatically when things go wrong. Their work necessarily involves prediction and they need support and training, not condemnation, for the work they do.

SEXUAL ABUSE

Sexual abuse is activity in which a child is used for adult arousal and of which secrecy is an essential component. Sexual touching, masturbation, the child witnessing adult sexual behaviour, seeing videos or magazines containing pornographic material – all constitute abuse. Its graver forms are oral sex, penetration and buggery. One adult and one child, or sometimes a group of adults and a number of children, are involved. Usually the abuser is known to the child and may be the father or stepfather, an older sibling, or relative or friend. Only rarely is serious abuse carried out by a woman. The victim may be a boy or a girl.

Much has been written about the two main approaches to understanding the problem, which are, respectively, either dysfunction within the family, or the ways in which men (and boys) express anger and inadequacy by using their power against those weaker than themselves. Family collusion, male power, the abuse itself, diagnosis and disclosure interviews, and counselling the adults involved are all important issues, but this section will be concerned primarily with the reaction of a sizeable group of unhappy children.

THE CHILDREN

The child, thinking that what is happening is normal, may enjoy the closeness, the rewards and the power that the sexual secret brings. There may well be natural physical pleasure. Any such reaction, though, will fit uneasily with the much more powerful feelings of isolation and guilt; of being different or dirty and of wishing the abuse would stop. Some feel they have cancer, that something has invaded them, and they attempt to alter this by continually washing in the hope that they will somehow get clean inside, too.

A large number experience fear and pain and, as with all abused children, the belief of their own badness and responsibility is very strong. Since it is inconceivable to blame a loved adult the child feels she must be at fault. Children under the age of four or five think that parents know everything, but for older children the trauma is compounded if the abuser is their father and they learn that their mother knew and did not protect them.

Because children react so differently to this experience we need to be open minded in thinking what it means to each individual child. Stereotyping is not helpful, although all children will be confused because a boundary has been crossed and, by losing trust in adults, their childhood has been spoiled.

Penny, the oldest girl in the family, had been sexually abused by a much-loved father from about the age of five. She learned very early on that he enjoyed her vivacity, and she enjoyed the closeness she had with him. To show that she hated the abuse would have risked losing her special place in the family. She dealt with the situation by fantasizing that she was two people and could remove her mind from her body. Thus somebody else was being abused while she remained the happy, smiling, coquettish little girl her father admired. The abuse stopped at puberty, as it often does and, after a stormy, promiscuous adolescence and an unsuccessful marriage to a much older man, she was helped to stop blaming herself and to shed tears for the unhappy child she had been.

A proportion of children have been abused by more than one person. Often this can be forgotten for years, but when it does become a conscious memory their distress can be devastating.

Perhaps it really was their fault? It is more likely that such a child develops a flirtatious manner to hide from herself that she had been abused and to protect the primary abuser, especially if it was her father. She could also be projecting an image of a vulnerable child from a family who were not too caring. If the parents, for what ever reason, were not aware of their child's distress and did not give the necessary warmth and protection, the child's need for a caring relationship would be obvious to anyone wanting to use her for their own gratification.

Rita came from such a family but reacted differently. She remembered the pleasure she had gained from spending the money her uncle gave her as part of the secret relationship, and she remembered that he alone made her feel she was valued. As a teenager, though, she was overwhelmed with guilt at the realization that she had accepted payment in return for the sexual relationship. She saw herself as dirty and disgusting, a prostitute who sold her body for money, and for many years could not believe that anyone would value her because, following this experience, she did not value herself.

Many children have told adults about what is happening but have not been believed. Others are burdened because they have not told, which is a difficult thing to do if you feel responsible. There may be some good reasons for keeping the secret. Perhaps they feel they can trust nobody, or will be called a liar. Children may be aware that their mother is vulnerable and needs to be protected from unpleasant facts. Mothers like this may not be able to react in a helpful way if they were abused themselves as children, for the whole problem is too painful to contemplate.

Another reason for staying silent is to protect the family from outside interference and to stay together. 'I will have to go to prison if you tell', is a powerful threat. Children may live under constant fear, either that their life is threatened or of some terrible punishment. One seven-year-old had lived in terror for years, believing the threat that Daddy would put her in the boiler if she made a fuss or told. 'The boiler fire needs stoking up', was his way of warning her.

Boys

Abused boys are usually less willing than girls to talk about their experiences. To do so might seem as if they were in a weak position, a role not reconcilable with masculinity. Fear might have made them petrified, unable to resist or respond. To make public the experience could be related to the fear of being thought homosexual, and if the abuse resulted in some pleasurable feelings this can cause tremendous guilt. But if we accept the prevailing view – that male abusers were themselves child victims – the most important task is to break this cycle. As with other situations, though, it must be remembered that not every abused boy grows up to be an abusing adult, because good experiences and caring relationships can help to change people's image of themselves and thus their behaviour.

Sometimes the abuser deliberately plans the abuse. He takes some time making friends with the boy he has chosen, then gradually makes sexual overtures to excite his victim and make him feel guilt and shame because the experience at first is secret and enjoyable. Because of these feelings the boy's silence is assured, and if the abuse continues he is in danger of having difficulty in forming relationships because of his damaged self-image.

Siblings

Possibly the next revelation to shock the nation will be the degree of incest which takes place between children who are related. The fact that the secret is hidden from the parents is a part of the relationship. Sometimes the siblings have turned to each other because parents have not provided warmth or excitement, or perhaps they comfort each other when their parents separate, as they feel their world is coming to an end. This close relationship highlights the feelings of being alive and needed by someone although there is often a component of aggression, too; a dominating older brother inducing fear in his younger brother or sister. Much about family life is still obscure.

Non-Abused Children

What do the non-abused children in the family feel? Relief that they were not the victim? Anger because they weren't favoured? Anger with the sibling who disclosed and upset everybody, or the perpetrator for doing it, or the mother for not stopping it? If the abuser is the father or stepfather and it is suspected that more than one child has been abused, then family therapy may be indicated, providing such intervention does not rule out the possibility of individual counselling or group work. Quite often the abuser is not faithful to one child, a possibility that is not always remembered. Sandra had been abused by her father for some years. She kept the secret until, when she was approaching puberty, he indicated that it would soon be her little sister's turn.

It was her maternal grandfather who had abused Emma while he was babysitting. Although he was not involved in any family meetings, it was important for the nuclear family to share their feelings about the event, but the mother also needed individual counselling to come to terms with what her father had done to her daughter. An added difficulty was that a younger, three-year-old sister who had not been abused could not understand why she was no longer allowed to see her favourite grandfather. But this is a typical situation; abuse usually has wide ramifications affecting many people.

Silences

All children, especially those who have known fear and lack confidence, will keep silent when they are disagreeing with a powerful adult (who can take this for acquiescence) because it is more comfortable for them or it is what they want to hear. This is important for child sexual-abusers – and counsellors – to remember. The different meanings silence can have are discussed in Chapter 9. If abuse is in question it can also mean 'yes' or 'no', 'I don't want to tell you'; 'That's too difficult for me to answer'; 'I didn't listen to the question'; 'If I told you, you wouldn't understand'; as well as more complicated attitudes: 'Think what you like, I don't care because you are just another Nosy Parker', or: 'I bet you would like to know the answer to that, but I'm not going to tell because I don't trust you'. Even what appears to be no behaviour gives a message.

MEN

The largest group of children are those abused by men, or older boys, known to them; the father being the most likely offender. The abuse is more likely to be a part of a relationship and not a one-off incident. The Butler-Sloss report (1988) found that sexual abuse occurs in all social classes, and while a small proportion of men are paedophiles, attracted only to children, the majority are thought to be active heterosexual men who, being immature, have a low level of control over their behaviour. It is equally relevant that many abusers have a history of violence or of sexual problems, the implication being that the personality difficulties began long before marriage and fatherhood.

Male abusers may have fantasies of women and children as possessions. Their distorted thinking, masking guilt and anxiety, makes them unable to accept that the child might in any way be harmed by the abuse and leads to the defence that the victim didn't protest, or even 'asked for it': 'she enjoyed it'; 'I was helping her grow up', they say, or: 'I was being a good, caring parent'. With this kind of thinking it is obvious that to stop a repetition of the crime requires a dramatic change and a great deal of skilled counselling.

WOMEN

A small portion of abusers are women; they may be mentally ill or lonely and use their child's body to comfort themselves. The abuse can take the form of intrusive inspections and cleansing or fondling in a way which crosses the generation boundary. The mother is failing to meet the child's need for respect and privacy and for freedom from being used for others' emotional satisfaction. A few women are involved in group sex with children but in any circumstances for women (rather than men) to harm their children is more upsetting to the general public because they have abdicated their traditional caring role. Fortunately the incidence of women abusers is small, though the harm they do to their children is great. Most were abused as children but, as with male abusers, there must be an army of women who were abused as children and do not continue the practice. Why not? Why do some women model themselves on the aggressor and some on the victim?

'A LIFE-SENTENCE'

Sexual abuse is a serious problem because of the distress and long-lasting effects on the child who has been betrayed: 'A life-sentence', were the words of a thirty-year-old child victim. It is damaging, too, because of the intensity of the experience. The trust children place in adults to protect them is shattered and they are forced to grow up sexually too soon. Guilt and the erosion of self-esteem are frequently the consequence, and every relationship can be affected adversely.

Some children come to terms with the trauma, but it is a long process. Daphne was abused, but recovered, partly because a friend of her parents who child-minded admitted the offences, but also because a sensitive social worker helped to free her from the burden of guilt. The scars it left, which took a long time to heal, were related to Daphne's dislike of her own teenage body and a fear of her growing maturity.

SEX RINGS

The first British sex ring to be uncovered was in 1984 in Leeds, but we still know little about children who are exploited in this way. In England the difficulties of helping boys who have taken part in sex rings has been analysed by Christopherson (1989). The numbers of children and adults can be very great – in one ring, up to 100 children. This poses a problem for the police investigating the offences and the social workers who aim to help the victims; the difficulties are compounded by fear and by the loyalty the children have to each other and to the group. But without appropriate treatment the majority will suffer some adverse effects and many may later identify with the abuser and thereby perpetuate the offence. Effective intervention is therefore essential.

CLEVELAND

In Cleveland, in the north of England, during the spring and summer of 1987, 157 instances of sexual abuse with children were diagnosed; twenty-six were deemed – some incorrectly, as it later transpired – to have been wrongly diagnosed and most of the others became subject to some form of state protection. A number were returned to their homes because the abuser had left. It is probable that the number wrongly diagnosed initially was quite small.

The subsequent enquiry, under Lord Justice Butler-Sloss (1988), revealed the fragmentation and inadequacy of the support system, but for the present purpose it was the new knowledge about the nature of the abuse which was important and which increased our knowledge of children subjected to this experience. Many of the Cleveland children were unexpectedly young, the average age being under seven years. The three-year-old baby with a sexually-transmitted disease, reported by Campbell (1988, p. 84), must have caused some people to modify their view of the problem. The youngest sexually abused child mentioned by Butler-Sloss was a six-week-old baby. Conventional wisdom had previously received another shock arising from the fact that for small girls vaginal abuse is difficult, but it is possible for both boys and girls to suffer anal abuse at a very young age. The implication of this observation by Drs Hobbs and Wynne (1986)[1] is that there were (and possibly still are) likely to be many undiagnosed abused boys.

DIAGNOSIS

Diagnosing the sexual abuse of girls and boys is complicated and controversial. Breaking down cultural barriers to increase the willingness of boys to disclose the abuse they have been subjected to is especially difficult, but nevertheless important. Depending on the passage of time and the nature of the abuse there may not be physical signs in the anal or genital areas, but the indications may be in family relationships: many children disclose then retract, sometimes repeatedly; some consistently deny the abuse and the pain; some do not disclose, but indicate by their sexual behaviour with other adults or children, or by their awareness of sexual practices. that abuse is likely to have occurred. Many show emotional distress. Rarely is one sign or symptom enough to diagnose child sexual-abuse with certainty.

The psychological indications, since Cleveland, are more widely recognised now: the isolated unhappy child, often friendless (if you allow people to get too close they might find out your secret); underfunctioning at school (it is difficult to concentrate), and those children who seem to take the role of victim with family and friends. Others have difficulty in sleeping (understandably – thoughts are worrying and confused and you never know whether someone will wake you up) and they behave in ways more appropriate to a younger child, as if emotional development has slowed down or stopped. The symptoms they display show some similarities with those displayed in post-trauma stress syndrome.

Finally, anger which cannot be expressed directly is turned inwards and is manifested in self-abuse, fears, phobias or feeding difficulties. Bizarre behaviour can be another indication. Anne, aged twelve, brought a doll to her exploratory sessions. She dressed and undressed it, alternately cuddled and spanked it and examined it for minute scratches. It was also used to divert any conversation which was painful for her. At this time she could not disclose the abuse, though she did later, and only showed by her behaviour that something was seriously wrong. Children who have not been abused may show some symptoms, but abused children are likely to display many of them and their conversation or actions may indicate a knowledge of sexual matters which could only come from first-hand knowledge.

If it is suspected, a full history of the child and the family and the family's reaction to the allegations might be revealing. The child's responses might indicate which part of the experience is most distressing. How does she react to the parents and how do they relate to her? From direct observation, how are the other children in the family behaving? Details of the parental history will be important in understanding the present. However, the likelihood of the abuser being another child or coming from outside the family must always be considered.

Helping the child feel safe enough to talk about what has happened requires a great deal of skill and will be the start of a long process of their ceasing to feel responsible and guilty and to stop self-blame; she must feel she is being believed. She might feel the responsibility of keeping the family together is hers and, even if she trusts someone enough to tell, her isolation can continue if siblings or mother blame her for breaking up the family. Often the mother's acceptance of her story and her support are crucial in making the child feel safe enough to disclose. The fear is that the consequences of telling will be more traumatic for the family than the abuse itself: painful questioning and long-delayed court appearances; the father in prison; the children sent away and the family unit broken. All are possibilities which might appear to outweigh the gains for the child.

COUNSELLING CHILDREN

Whether the concern is with disclosure or counselling, timing is important. So, too, is the provision of a place where the child can feel safe, have a degree of control over the interview and be believed. Rarely do children lie about abuse. They need to be reassured that they will not be blamed and that it is not their fault. It will probably be some time before the child feels safe enough to share the full extent of the trauma she has experienced.

Some interesting work has been done with children's groups, the aim being to reduce the child's feeling of isolation and build up trust in adults. Children can gain confidence and learn what is 'good touch' and what is not, and in a caring and supportive atmosphere the full story can be told.

Whether in groups or individually, the counsellor will be in direct contact with the child's pain and the hate she feels for everyone, especially herself. These feelings may be directed towards the counsellor, but only when this phase is reached, as in bereavement counselling, will there be the hope of growth, maturity and happiness, but it is a long hard road for all concerned and it is very easy to be taken in by the child who has made progress while leaving the core of the pain untouched.

The strength of children's resilience never ceases to amaze those who deal with children subjected to torment and terror while growing up, whatever form it takes. Too many children today are being used emotionally by adults, and their need for unconditional loving and respect has been forgotten by parents concerned to put their own needs first. Children's need for affection and physical contact is not sexual and should never be exploited as such.

7 DIVORCE AND CHILDREN

CHILDREN'S REACTIONS

'I'm like Humpty Dumpty: no-one can put me together again.' So said an eight-year-old girl whose parents had recently divorced. She felt responsible because her father, shortly before he left, had been cross with her for not feeding her pet rabbit. She believed that it was both his anger with her and her unspoken angry retaliatory feelings against him which had caused him to leave. After his departure her guilt and anxiety about the future were very much in her mind but the parents were so preoccupied with their own feelings that they were unable to appreciate her distress, believing that silence meant she had got over it.

Whatever the age of the child at the time of separation, four emotions are generally present in differing degrees. The first and most pervasive is *sadness* related to loss of a loved parent and perhaps other relatives in the family. This feeling is akin to mourning and is often accompanied by waves of loneliness and yearning. Also present will be *anger* at being so impotent and unable to change the situation. *Anxiety* may relate to past or future: children are not sure whether they were in some way responsible for what happened and they can also be worried about what changes will occur because, from the child's viewpoint, there seems to be very little which will be better. The fourth emotion is *confusion* about why parents need to divorce: at least one parent perceives it as an absolute necessity, the child sees it as a deliberate choice. Divided loyalty and the need to protect parents make it difficult for her to ask questions about these feelings, especially if she suspects the answers are not what she wants to hear.

Not a few children are relieved when the anger and discord have ended. Different feelings will be paramount at different times but whatever the quality of life had been prior to divorce, and however unsatisfactory the care, most children do not want their parents to separate. They have an identity within the family and have learnt some survival strategies in order to deal with the familiar rows and tensions. The unknown holds greater fears.

Young Children

Separation from a father may be more traumatic for a small boy of around three years than at later ages. This is the age when his feelings about his parents are changing. He is very close to his mother: 'I'm going to marry Mummy when I grow up', he says. Daddy is loved and wanted but is also a rival for Mummy; if Daddy leaves he has been victorious but Daddy might want revenge. Monsters and vicious animals invade his sleep and sometimes spill over into daytime activities as well, especially if contact is broken. But another aspect of this stage of development is that he is starting to give up being Mummy's baby to become Daddy's little boy, a process made easier if he has a model with which to identify, to help with his maleness.

The little three-year-old girl can become equally anxious. She was going to marry Daddy when she grew up but he didn't want her and has left, presumably because of something she has done. Contact and reassurance that he still loves her even if he lives somewhere else is very important for her future image of herself.

Those who work with divorcing families hear many stories of children staring out of the window for long periods, yearning for Daddy. The child may be thinking that if the impossible can happen, and Daddy really has left me, perhaps Mummy will leave too, then who will get my dinner? Anxiety may be shown by clinging behaviour, fear of many things and often difficulty in sleeping, while the anger is expressed in apparently incomprehensible outbursts. The more disturbed child will lose all confidence and become a sad onlooker, watching the world go by, isolated and unhappy, thumb in mouth, detached, fearful, desperate for love but unable to ask for it or respond when it is offered because trust has gone.

Children under about five years do not understand what divorce means, although they do understand that Daddy has left, and, as all small children do, believe that they must be responsible, probably because they were naughty. Sometimes the sadness they feel is overwhelming, defying words. That something can be for ever is inconceivable for small children: Daddy will come back when he has done what he has to do. Their belief in magic sadly doesn't work, so for these young children the acceptance of the separation being permanent can take years and last long after their dream that one day Mummy and Daddy will get married again is relinquished.

'He's too young to understand', adults say, to reassure themselves – but he is not too young to feel lonely and abandoned.

Middle Childhood

Children of junior-school age have more sense of reality but also react with tremendous sadness and often guilt. For those who find difficulty in thinking of anything else, progress at school suffers. Some children, though, are able to separate school from home and, in an attempt to prove to themselves that they can succeed somewhere, do well. They find the routine of school life reassuring and safe.

They may have difficulty in leaving home to attend school because of anxiety about the remaining parent. Often these are first-born or only children, who, taking a protective parenting role, use mental energy which would be better spent in maturation.

Generation boundaries can be crossed in other ways, as when a parent treats the child as the absent parent. 'You are the man of the house now', can be a tremendous burden on a small child who has enough problems of his own to deal with besides being given such inappropriate responsibility. For a lone mother to share her bed with a growing son for a long time may also add to confusion, though at the time of separation parent and child will need extra support and comfort from each other. An older child may also fall into the role of parent to his younger siblings.

The inability of a child in middle childhood to accept the situation causes some to do what they can to effect a reconciliation. One way might be to try to unite parents in their concern for her own health, so psychosomatic illness such as unexplained tummy pains is one unconscious weapon to use. Failure to take care is another. Ian fell out of a tree and broke his leg; Sally scalded herself severely with boiling water: two desperately sad children, unconsciously trying to unite their parents in joint concern. Alternatively, there may be the feeling that if no one is bothered about you then it is not worth keeping yourself safe.

Other children behave badly in an attempt to unite their parents, using many unconscious behaviours to this end. Straightforward mourning for the departed parent is usually private, many children feeling that with all the anger around they alone hold the sadness for the family, in secret.

We know something of children's reaction to divorce from an American study. [1] Boys between the ages of six and eight were most devastated by their father's departure, being more conscious of sorrow than any other group and frequently sobbing or having bizarre fantasies of being abandoned or being without food. The nine- and ten-year-olds were more contained. They felt more shame about their situation and were concerned to hide their distress under restless activity. However, they were more likely to take sides and express anger against the 'bad' one, especially if this was the parent of the same sex who had been a model for them but now leaves them bewildered and bereft.

Adolescence

As adolescence approaches, moral dilemmas arise. Who is right and who is wrong? I want to live with my father/mother but he/she caused the divorce so it wouldn't be fair to the other parent. There is some evidence that adolescent girls are especially vulnerable to the breakup of their parents' marriage at a time when they are trying to sort out their own emotional life and are wondering about forming their own sexual relationships.

Older adolescents may be more detached because they are aware that many of their contemporaries are in a similar situation, although they may wonder, as do many younger children, if they will be able to make a stable marriage themselves in the future. Their anchor has gone; their childhood has ended before they are ready. The anguish of these teenagers who have lost their secure base is intense, despite the compensation of greater independence. It can feel wrong to them: parents leaving adolescents is not the right way round; they should be leaving parents. This reversal of the expected can leave them feeling depressed, lonely and occasionally suicidal: you say you love me but you don't care about my life at all; you have betrayed me.

Nor is it unusual for adolescents, and sometimes younger children to change their minds, finding the first parent they live with too restrictive. After moving, they discover that this parent also is not the liberal person they had imagined. Is there nowhere I belong? Is anybody responsible for me?

All Children

Some reactions occur at any age. Development can appear to stop, as if the next stage is too difficult; children may regress, possibly to get attention but more likely as a retreat into a time when life was straightforward. Terry, a sad little six-year-old, repeatedly drew tearful owls in his therapy sessions. He and his mother were both upset by his reverting to bed-wetting. When he accepted the inevitability of his parents' separation and found his worst fears were not realized because he still saw Daddy, the symptom disappeared and before long he drew cars and aeroplanes.

Coping strategies will be needed to help a child trying to deal with the pain of separation from a loved parent. Feeling different from other children and powerless to prevent such an awful thing happening are likely to be present as well as the sadness and anxiety. But sometimes they can contribute to the stress, when their helplessness leads them to gain power by manipulating their parents. 'I saw Daddy in a big new car'; or, 'Mummy didn't come home until midnight last night', are more obvious attempts to play one parent against the other.

Obviously not all respond with the same intensity; sensitive children, attuned to atmosphere and aware of adults' actions, can act as a shield for other children in the family, protecting them from some of the stress. The trauma will be less severe where children are supported by a caring family and friends, but parental concern for them, before separation and during it, is of the greatest significance. One or two things will help the children, notably telling them clearly and honestly what is taking place in a way they understand. Equally important, they should know that thought has been given to their feelings about where they will live and how the relationship with both parents will continue. They should know that both parents are concerned about their welfare and, despite no longer loving each other, still love them; unfortunately, though it has to be recognised that several parents do not, in fact, have a caring relationship with their children. Much can be done to lessen the trauma. However, it is all too easy to increase it, and it is not helpful, for instance, to use a child of any age as a messenger, spy or go-between.

Parents who have been involved in legal battles are in a more difficult position because the adversarial system highlights the differences between them. Battlelines are drawn: I am right and you are wrong; I behaved reasonably but you told lies and are not a good parent. Angry words can spill over onto the child in a destructive way at this juncture in the divorce process.

What is most helpful is for the parents to remain friendly, at least when the children are around. Often what is difficult is to accept is the spouse's new partner because of the fear that your child will have a new parent who might take your place in the child's affections. Rejection, jealousy and anger are powerful, primitive feelings which can override the parent's wish to be reasonable in the interests of the child.

If a child shows she is distressed or behaves in a way which causes concern it may be related to divorce, but not necessarily so. There are many hurdles to negotiate while growing up and problems may well be related to events quite apart from separated parents. Children of divorced parents are not the only ones who manifest behaviour disorders or exhibit anxiety.

WAR BETWEEN TWO PARENTS OR PEACE WITH ONE?

Parents and others often believe that it is better for children to be brought up by one parent in a non-stressful home than by two quarrelling parents. This, though, is not the opinion of most of the fifty children in a British survey conducted to test this piece of conventional wisdom;[2] they preferred the unhappy marriage to divorce, a conclusion confirmed by the American research referred to above. The children's perception was of a situation neither better nor worse than that of other families around them, whereas the American researchers frequently wondered why the parents took so long to end a relationship in which both were 'demeaned, neglected and abused'. Anyone who listens to children hears of their being torn apart by the rows – lying under the bedclothes at night, stiff and still, trying to hear and not to hear the angry words from downstairs, praying the row or fighting will soon end – or of living with the nightly fear that Daddy would come home drunk and violent. Scenes like these, frightening and horrible though they are, become an accepted part of life for children and, so the majority of them apparently believe, they are better than having separated parents.

This is the child's preference, but there is another dimension to the problem. It is more likely that children who display conduct disorders come from homes where hostility and conflict are the norm. It is family discord which increases the risk of behavioural difficulties, not how many parents a child lives with. All too often, antagonism between separated parents continues, sometimes for years, to the detriment of the children.

The complexities of this issue need disentangling to determine which factors counteract the bad effects. The latter are not irreversible; a good relationship with one parent may counterbalance a bad relationship with the other and so reduce the damage to the child. Balance, though, is hard to judge in advance of divorce, for some of the consequences – notably low income – can affect the child for a long time, resulting in a lower standard of living. Relationships, too, can be tense: perhaps the mother, upset and angry by the divorce, manages the children less well than formerly. The boys in the family, missing their dad, can become difficult and defiant. Fortunately the evidence suggests that after about two years the situation begins to improve (Wolkind & Rutter, 1985).

Divorce following disclosure of sexual abuse raises problems requiring specialist knowledge and will not be discussed here.

AT THE TIME OF SEPARATION

Awareness of the effect of separation on children is increasing, yet, at the time it takes place, parents understandably tend to be so preoccupied with their own feelings that they are unable to empathize with the child. Two very caring divorced parents were surprised and shocked when asked about this and admitted that they had no idea what their daughter had felt. Then they remembered that one night, just before the actual separation, they had found her sobbing uncontrollably, something they had both 'forgotten' for four years.

Some children (especially the eldest one in the family) know that Mummy has a boyfriend or Daddy isn't too bothered about the family at present, but for others divorce can come as a complete surprise, like a thunderstorm on a fine day. The child in the first situation might have picked up signals which alerted her to impending change, though sometimes the fear of what might happen is worse than reality. In the second situation a child will need a great deal of sensitive support to come to terms with what is, in her eyes, a disastrous event. Fortunately, children are usually forgiving, providing someone is sensitive to their feelings.

Amid all the upset and trauma, the school is sometimes not informed, an omission which can have unfortunate consequences. Children show distress in many ways, one being uncooperative behaviour at school, and another, an inability to concentrate; both cause them to fall behind academically. A sympathetic approach by the school is very important for the child.

It can be next to impossible for small children to imagine the unthinkable – that Mummy and Daddy will not be living together any more – and the question, sometimes unasked, is: What will happen to me? From the child's point of view the statistics are grim; the British study mentioned above found that one-third of absent parents lose contact straight away, and within five years another third will have lost touch.

The difficulties of sustaining such a relationship are considerable. Some parents lose contact to protect themselves from the pain of seeing their child for brief periods only; others find intermittent meetings make it hard to relate to a growing child. Material considerations may hinder contact, including distance and lack of money. Parental attitudes may clash, resulting in increased difficulties in maintaining the relationship. Not all parents feel affection for their child, or what they had cannot survive the diminished contact. Some enjoy the idea of being a parent and would maintain, with truth, that they love their child, but the actual demands of the relationship – the closeness, the time and patience necessary for good parenting – are not wanted or enjoyed.

TELLING THE CHILDREN

It is harmful for children to have to find out what is going on by trying to make sense of overheard conversations. Something adults can't talk about must be very dreadful. For some weeks, June thought her absent father, who had formed another relationship, was working away from home. She was distressed because he had not said goodbye to her; his avoidance of pain was interpreted by her as an indication that he did not really love her. She learned the truth by overhearing her mother's telephone conversation with a solicitor. Terrible anger with both parents plus her sense of loss led to her losing all trust in adults and caused serious emotional problems.

For young children, the fact that what is happening is not their fault has to be repeated until it is believed. This is easier to accept in families where children have been told about things honestly and have had the experience of being listened to in the past. Two twins aged ten were having to face the fact that their mother was leaving home. Because they had been treated with respect and their feelings considered, they could ask questions and be slightly comforted. They understood that Mummy did love them but at present she was too upset to keep in touch with them except by phone, but she hoped this situation would not last long and things would improve. Although distressed, they did not loss their trust in adults. It is too late to relate to children in a different way at a time of crisis.

Parents are often concerned about what to tell the children at the time of divorce. Neither 'we couldn't get on together', nor 'Daddy doesn't love us', are helpful. The impact of being told, without further explanation, that 'Daddy and Mummy don't love each other any more although they will always love you', can be shattering for a child who, until this moment, believed that love was something that lasted for ever. Is it because someone has been naughty that you stop loving them?

Ideally parents should talk to the children together, explaining what has happened and what is likely to happen and assuring them of their continued love. Children should know that the difficulties are between adults, not about them. The message, to be repeated many times, is that it is all right to love both parents; children don't have to choose between them. Handling the telling badly can have long-lasting effects. A mother aged thirty, whose marriage was in crisis, said with tears in her eyes that her parents had split up when she was fifteen and she was still resentful.

Unfortunately, fathers who have left the family sometimes find the task of telling the children too painful and leave the mother to do her best. In a well-intentioned attempt to protect them from seeing their father as less than perfect she may blame his new partner for his departure, but in the long term it will not be in the children's best interests; if this person subsequently becomes their stepmother it will increase their difficulties in getting to know her and could jeopardize their relationship with their father.

Children might be able to understand that they have changed from how they were, say, two years ago. Adults, too, can change; sometimes in ways that cause them to grow apart from each other. When Mummy and Daddy got married they loved each other and thought they always would; there were lots of good things about this loving – one of them, having children – but once they stop loving each other it becomes difficult to live together and to be happy. They tried very hard but did not succeed. This is sad for parents, too, but they hope that, by splitting up, everybody will be happier in the long run. If, as is often the case, one parent has fallen in love with someone else, then the task of telling the children is harder, but it has to be done with as much understanding of their feelings as possible. As has been said before, it is not what has happened but how children interpret events which is important.

If the matter is not discussed, children can be anxious about the possibility of parents not loving them for ever, and then what would happen? This confusion, arising from use of the word 'love' for two different feelings with some common elements, is difficult for parents to explain and requires some elaboration.

LOVING

Normally, in marriage the love that one adult has for another is based initially on sexual attraction. Implicit in it is the hope of a deep relationship which involves both sharing and companionship, but also a respect for the other's individuality and independence. Each will expect to be valued for what they are as well as what they do, and to feel special despite being less than perfect. Mutual trust is also needed, as well as giving and receiving support when things go wrong.

Love between a parent and child is also likely to be about each making the other feel good but the expectations are different. The child wants unconditional love from the parent – the feeling that whatever she does, she will still be loved. That this is so is revealed by the intensity of feeling for a parent even among those who are badly treated: they never give up hope that one day things will change and they will be loved. Consequently, most children want to please their parents and, if they have been treated with respect, respect their parents in return.

The love of a parent for a child is more likely to be permanent; it is less complex than that between adults because it contains a strong element of being part of each other and usually has lasted as long as the child has lived. Incorporated in it is a feeling of responsibility, and pleasure in the different stages the child reaches. Change is welcomed because it represents growing maturity. There may be the feeling that the child belongs to this family, she is the future. Unfortunately, some adults who have loving feelings for their child are unable to show they care, either because they are embarrassed or feel they might be taken advantage of. This is a sad situation; love can be shown to a child in many ways besides words. It is important to convey to children in intelligible terms the feeling that you are glad they are around, pleased at their successes, sympathetic when things go wrong and prepared to give time to them with enjoyment.

Parents are quite often asked: 'Who do you love the best; me or my sister/brother?'. An easy answer is: 'I love you both the same', but this is not what the child wants to hear and it is not entirely true because loving is complex and entwined with other feelings. Love for a child can include a feeling of pride or concern, or the child is enjoyed for her sense of humour, her enthusiasm or her warmth. All can be loved but in different ways. The message all children want to hear is: I love you because you are you and very special to me. If a child really believes that, then she will not be concerned about making comparisons with the other children in the family – she knows that there is enough love to go round for them all to feel special.

AFTER THE SEPARATION

CONCILIATION

When parents divorce, local authorities have a duty under the Children Act 1989 to protect and promote the welfare of children in need, and courts are enjoined to pay particular attention to a child's wishes and feelings. The Act further states that a court shall not make an order unless it considers that doing so would be better for the child than making no order at all. Normally, both parents will have a duty to look after their children and both will share parental responsibility (although if unmarried, a court order or parental responsibility agreement will be necessary for legal parental responsibility). Of the many changes enacted in this piece of legislation, these are the most relevant to the issue of conciliation (now increasingly referred to as mediation).

One consequence is that arrangements regarding a child's contact with both parents are more likely to be the outcome of a voluntary agreement between parents rather than, as formerly, a decision made by the court. Conciliation, based on co-operation and compromise rather than confrontation, is increasingly important and is likely to be better for the children.

Different schemes operate in different parts of the country, but in-court conciliation, carried out by Court Welfare Officers working in Civil Units, is available in courts concerned with divorce matters. Couples are seen while at the court, and an attempt is made to help them come to an acceptable agreement; around half do so successfully. The remainder may be offered further conciliation and, if agreement cannot be reached, a welfare inquiry is prepared for the court.

Some areas have a Voluntary Conciliation Service which, using experienced volunteers, provides confidential meetings to help the couple come to an agreement about issues concerning the children. Conciliation is a good way of proceeding because decisions reached by compromise avoid court proceedings in this often very painful area, thus saving a great deal of time. In some places, independent services affiliated to the National Family Conciliation Council have been set up, though their brief is usually wider than concern with the children.[3] One aspect of the work which should be extended is to offer children the opportunity to talk about their feelings in confidence, always making sure they know that even though their views are important, decisions are made by parents, not them.

In parental interviews, emphasis is placed not on the marriage or what has happened in the past, but on the future. In confidential discussions parents can be encouraged to set aside their own feelings and focus on the best interests of their children. Many find this difficult because the continuing anger, masking deep hurt about what happened in the marriage, is overwhelming. Too often, what should be an end to a relationship is very different. The ex-husband drives past his ex-wife's house and notes the car standing in the drive; the ex-wife is curious about her ex-husband's new partner; the notion that indifference is the opposite of love does not appear to apply at this time.

Divorce is a process and, as in all significant relationships, feelings change. It is as if parents are climbing a ladder; to get to the top they take painful steps – denial, sadness, and terrible anger, which can feel like madness may be among them. Near the top is a step called acceptance, but the top step, from which they can see the future, is called independence. Then there is belief in themselves with gives a new courage. It is time to make changes.[4]

Evidence suggests that those children who do best have had as much as possible of what is familiar kept intact. Thus, on balance they are less distressed if they continue to live in their own home, attend the same school, and engage in the same activities. It is even more important for both parents to be interested and involved in their children's growing up.

CONTACT

The child's picture of herself as unwanted and unloved is confirmed if, for instance, birthdays are not acknowledged. While some mothers want the father's contact (previously known as access) to cease, believing that the upset is not worth the effort of arranging meetings and opening old wounds, others empathize with the child to the extent of sending cards and presents 'from Daddy' when Daddy is only concerned with a new life and does not want to be reminded of a painful past. If clear-cut arrangements concerning contact can be made as soon as possible, based on the best compromise for everyone, and both divorced parents see their task as helping the other to be as good a parent as possible, then the psychological damage to the children involved will be minimal. The situation calls for honesty by all concerned because parenting is about responsibility which cannot be evaded without tremendous damage to a dependent child.

The experience of contact is not easy for fathers without their own home and perhaps in financial difficulties. Where do you take children whom you do not really know and who are changing rapidly, when McDonald's is boring and it's a wet Sunday afternoon and you've already been to the museum twice this year and everything else is closed or too expensive? A few enlightened authorities and voluntary organisations have opened Contact Centres where the non-custodial parent and child can meet and develop their relationship together. This is infinitely better than the idea of loving the child without the contact, or having to meet in an unsuitable place. The visits are not without difficulty for some fathers because of conflicting emotions; not surprisingly, some find it easier to show love by providing sweets or toys (although they know that what is really needed is a pair of shoes).

The children want the parent's time; they want assurance, backed by some demonstration, not just words, that even if they do not meet very often they will always have a very special place in their father's thoughts. The situation can be easier if there is a relative's or grandparent's house where the children can be taken, providing they are not ignored in the adult conversation or merely expected to watch the television and 'be good'. Contact can be successful if properly planned to include time for activity, quiet (that is, television), talk and, if possible, something familiar and something new.[5]

The feelings of each child in the family need to be considered separately. One may feel sorry for the absent parent and express the sympathy for him or her, thus freeing the other children from the responsibility of maintaining the relationship; another may be the depository for the anger of all the children. Sometimes children say they do not want to see the other parent because the fear of upsetting the parent they live with is too great. If I enjoy being with Daddy too much, the child thinks, I am being disloyal to Mummy. In some families a child is identified with the absent parent and receives all the negative feelings which belong to that parent. It is important to appreciate that each child feels differently about the parents after the divorce from how she felt before the separation. It is too easy and often wrong to believe that the more vocal one is speaking for all.

The non-custodial parent with contact has many difficulties. Frequently, fathers resent the time-restrictions imposed on them.

They would like to take the child out when it is convenient for them, arguing that this should be their right as fathers. Having to wait until the next prescribed visiting time is a reminder of their powerlessness and can feel like punishment.

After the initial adaptation to change there can be some gains for the child. If the mother has custody, some children see more of their father on their contact visits than they ever did before, and a new, closer, relationship can develop. Perhaps before the separation childcare was left to the mother, for whatever reason, now it can be shared. Divorce gives the opportunity for a new start, something schools can help with by remembering to involve both parents in the school activities, providing this is done with tact. Each parent sees the children differently and each child sees the parents as individuals with their own personalities and interests.

Children may benefit in other ways. The likelihood is that they will become more self-reliant and, if their own have been respected, will gain more understanding of other people's feelings, learning, for example, that parents, too, appreciate some sign that they are valued by their children.

Some children, on returning home from a contact visit, are rude and difficult, so much so that the parent they live with wonders if the visits should stop or become less frequent. This may not be the right thing, depending on the meaning of the behaviour. The belief that the child has been 'spoilt' and resents the return to discipline and order is not normally the whole picture. For the child, the visits are a reminder that parents are separate, that loyalties are difficult and it is easier to be angry than sad. Moreover, bad behaviour stops the questioning about what has been happening and avoids the pain and sadness. Another explanation relates to the child feeling she must control the end of the day, especially if she has been 'good' all day. This can be relevant in other situations, too, when a child has had an enjoyable time but has to spoil the ending by unacceptable behaviour. These are some of the ways the child is trying to deal with emotional stress; to increase the visits is sometimes helpful, but the best way to find out is to discuss the problem with the child at a suitable time.

NO CONTACT?

Children have a right to know both parents and except in a very few instances this right should be respected. If this does not happen there is a risk that the absent parent will be idealised and so affect the child's later relationships adversely. Nor it is unknown for the custodial parent to be blamed later for depriving the child of the missing parent.

The exceptions should include fathers whose behaviour has caused their children great fear. Michael's and Jenny's father would become very violent after drinking and had a history of hitting both wife and children. After the mother left him, taking her children, he harassed them continually and on one occasion tried to break down the door of their new home with an axe. Other frightening incidents followed and it was thought that the terrified children would be better off not seeing their father. The older one said he wanted his mummy to find a 'gentle' daddy. Attempts to help the father refrain from doing his small children 'significant harm', using the words of the Children Act 1989, had failed.

If a husband was violent to his wife prior to divorce, will he be violent to his small daughter when she is disobedient? This is what many mothers fear and is a problem which causes great stress. There is no single answer. It is also difficult to decide whether a parent is causing an unacceptable level of emotional harm to a child. An instance of such harm is one who continually denigrates the other parent in front of the child, thus causing a division of loyalties which can have crippling emotional consequences.

It may be that the child does not want contact with the parent because there has never been a relationship between them, or because the child has been exploited by the parent. This is a compelling reason for the child's feelings to be heard and taken into consideration when decisions involving contact are taken, provided the views expressed are the child's and not the custodial parents'.

FATHERS WITH CUSTODY

Most children of divorced parents (more than 1.5 million in England and Wales) live with their mother, but about one in seven with their father. Some problems are common to both, such as making a satisfactory social life for themselves. Another difficulty separated parents face is having to accept, perhaps for the first time, that a growing part of their child's life is separate from them and they will play little or no part in it.

Dealing with daughters can present problems. Tilley was being cared for by her father, her mother having left for a man who was much more fun. On the threshold of adolescence she looked increasingly like her attractive mother, of whom she was a constant reminder to her father – reactivating the anger and hurt he had felt when she left. These unconscious feelings relating to her mother caused him to forbid Tilley to go out in the evenings with friends, so jeopardizing their previous warm relationship.

MOTHERS AS LONE PARENTS

Mothers left to bring up a family single-handed have a difficult problem which may be compounded by loneliness and poverty. Its extent is shown by the statistic that three-quarters of them received Income Support in 1992. If they have a job, child-minding can be fraught with anxiety. Those without friends or extended family can be doubly burdened, and may become quite seriously depressed and unable to meet the emotional needs of the children satisfactorily. In these circumstances, especially if the divorce was not wanted, self-confidence can plummet.

Using a son as a confidant – a fairly common pattern – may help the mother but certainly not the son; in contrast, just as Tilley had an inadvertent adverse effect upon her father, so some mothers find their son a constant reminder of the man who caused their predicament, especially if his acting-out behaviour keeps alive the 'bad' father for both of them. Without a model, a boy can grow up believing that women are all powerful, with the corollary that men are inferior – not a good basis on which to form male identity. Having other adult males around helps the child to form a more balanced view.

The mother on her own may have to accept that the children do not see their father in the same way as she does. The husband who sleeps around or gambles all the family money away may be seen in negative terms by a wife who has lost all trust and love for him, unlike his children who see him as the best dad in the world. However hard she tries, it is difficult not to let her anger erupt in the children's hearing from time to time, but it is important that the children do not hear repeatedly that their father is a bad man; nothing could be more damaging to their self-confidence. How can you be OK if even one of your parents is a bad person? You must be bad too.

Despite the received opinion about single-parent families, the majority of mothers react in ways helpful to the children. Most eventually find the courage to start a satisfactory new life, accepting that mistakes were made but, having worked through the different stages of denial, anger and depression, they have survived the experience. They face the future with a confidence which helps them and, indirectly, their children by freeing them from the sense of responsibility. Now Mum is strong enough to look after us. The worst is over; we will survive and manage better than before. We can start enjoying life again.

A word of caution, though. Alison's mother very sensitively told her daughter that one day it was likely that she would marry Ken, her boyfriend, whom Alison liked. She was very surprised at her daughter's distress upon hearing the news and presumed it was related to Alison's feelings about her father. Only later did Alison tell her that marriages meant anger and unhappiness and she did not want that experience to be repeated for her or her mother. Parents have to be wary of jumping to conclusions, as mistakes result if incorrect assumptions are made about children's thinking.

CHILDREN WITH STEP-PARENTS

Many different permutations in stepfamilies and the relations within them can be set aside in favour of a discussion focused on the children involved and their feelings.

In an unbroken family every member has a memory which stretches over years to include important events, happy times and tragedies which add up to a family identity. All of its members share myths and beliefs about themselves and they all know what is acceptable behaviour and what is not, from small matters such as table manners to moral standards. In brief, they have a shared image about themselves which has evolved over time.

The stepfamily is far more complicated; to establish accepted family rules takes time and is made more difficult by feelings of guilt, rivalry and jealousy between its members. Each child has a history, a past, which is not shared by everyone. Each brings expectations about the future which are not necessarily shared by the others.

It can be difficult for adults to understand the strength of a child's loyalty to both parents. Vicky liked the person who was shortly to become her stepmother but refused to be a bridesmaid at the wedding, despite great pressure. She would not say why because she could not share her real feelings. How could she forget the last nine years and pretend she wasn't sad? How could she say that even at this time she still had not given up hope that Daddy would come home again? And how could she say that to be part of such an occasion would make her feel intensely disloyal to her mother? She also felt that if her stepmother-to-be had any idea of the strength of her feelings she could not possibly like her or want her.

When a new family involving children is formed, there will be hope of happiness, a new beginning and the expectation that things will be better than before. What can be forgotten is that everyone involved also brings some sense of loss and often failure. Parents believe that the new family will be better for the children. They may nurse a hope that they will be exactly like a family where the children live with their natural parents. Some may be misguided enough to believe that the child wants to be rescued.

Too often, the reality is very different. Parents may think that their love for each other will be strong enough to overcome whatever difficulties present themselves, but the children's perception is often one of sadness for the loss of their previous family life and anger that they were powerless to do anything about it. Not a few will have feelings of guilt. Were they to blame? Could they have done anything to stop the breakup? If they do not blame themselves then someone else must be responsible and the obvious person is the step-parent.

A newly-wed, well-intentioned parent may feel that the second marriage is a new start and therefore it is better for the child to forget the natural parent and become part of the new family. 'She is happy', says the mother, 'and she calls her stepfather "Daddy". It is better for her to forget her real Dad'. This solution means the child has to deny half of her heritage and all of her previous life experience. She quickly learns from non-verbal cues that her real father cannot be mentioned. If there is no proper explanation, what is a child to think?

Either Dad doesn't want her or half of her is too awful to be talked about. She does not know that her mother is not secure enough in the new relationship to be able to consider her needs and to appreciate that, whether the child sees him or not, her dad is an integral part of herself and is likely to remain so for a very long time. As a consequence, difficulties may arise when a baby is born, or at adolescence. In fact, it is perfectly possible for a child to belong to two or sometimes more families perfectly happily if the adults concerned can balance past and present; the past must not be ignored but neither must it dominate the present.

From the child's point of view there is likely to be loss following separation of parents: loss of the companionship of a loved parent; loss of the undivided attention of the parent they are living with because affections are shared, the child being excluded for part of the time. The list might be extended to include loss of home, school, grandparents and other caring relatives, friends, income level and the security the family unit previously provided. If there are stepchildren in the new family there may be loss of previous position: the eldest; the youngest; the only girl, and so on, and space may be inadequate.

There may, of course, be gains: extra relatives with different interests, or the experience of belonging to a large family. The child might have seen her parents as one unit, but now they are two different people who are aware of different aspects of her, too. After the initial stresses, jealousies and grieving have been worked through, the new step-parent may also be seen differently. The increased independence which results from the change can be a bonus, as is the freedom from living in a household of tension and strife. There may be a long-term benefit too; a loving adult relationship where people are concerned to make others happy may be a new experience which can serve as a model for the future.

STEP-PARENTS

Step-parents have to give up the idea that they are substitute parents. They are not, because there is no shared history, and to achieve a warm relationship can easily take many years. The difficulty of doing so is implicit in the problem of what the step-parent should be called. What he or she can actually be, as distinct from the mode of address, is more important, for the step-parent can be another caring person in the child's life who can show kindness, give warmth and express interest – but this is not easy to achieve.

Stepmothering is a particularly difficult relationship, one not usually seen positively. No little girl says: 'I'm going to be a stepmother when I grow up', unless, possibly, she is being brought up by one.[6] The stepmother is trying to care for the children, make a good marital relationship, and preserve her own individuality and interests. The task is to harmonize the three roles and, in addition, she might also have to come to terms with her (very natural) jealousy of the first wife. It is not an easy situation.

Given the complexity of the demands on a stepmother it is not surprising that she should blame herself when things go wrong. In reality, all people in her position will have mixed feelings, some loving, some negative, for their stepchildren. Resentment may arise when the problems seem unsoluble, although the child's difficult behaviour could easily be age-appropriate and not related to being a stepchild. This is a time of tiredness and frustration, of feeling useless and resenting the lack of personal space. She is probably trying to do the impossible and is in need of help and support from her new partner, for what is absolutely crucial is that, as in all families, the key relationship must be between the parents, and the children must be aware of this.

It is often easier to be a stepfather because the relationship is not so intense and it may be easier to find shared activities. One danger is that he may have been trapped into disciplining the stepchildren before trust and warmth have developed, to the detriment of the relationship. Many, whether fathers or stepfathers, are reluctant to be involved in emotional issues, opting out rather than giving essential support, and failing to appreciate the need for honest discussion about all stressful matters, the trivial as well as the important.

A stepfather may have a fantasy about being the child's real parent and may find it difficult to understand how a child can continue to love a parent who, in his eyes, was unsatisfactory. He has to accept the child's need for the natural parent, whatever his own picture of that person, and respect the child's feelings. This may be complicated by feelings of rivalry if the child looks like the absent parent and is a reminder of the new spouse's previous sexual relationship. It was particularly difficult for one stepfather whose stepson had inherited a vivid shock of red hair from his dad.

Boundaries between a stepfamily and a natural family must be respected. When Robert went to spend a weekend with his father and stepmother, his mother asked them not to give him any treats because he had been stealing. In the event the father took his child to a football match, feeling that his ex-wife should respect his separateness.

THE CHILDREN'S RELATIONSHIP WITH
THEIR STEPMOTHER

Undoubtedly, some children settle down immediately in their new family and show little signs of difficulty, but another pattern, for girls in particular, is to see the stepmother as a rival for the father's affections, an interloper who has ruined her life. Among the strategies she can use to deal with this is to ignore the stepmother completely, making her feel superfluous. Although Helen had been told by her stepmother that they were going on holiday to Wales the next month, she asked her father if he had arranged a holiday for them.

She refused the food her stepmother had cooked and would make reference to past jokes and events: 'Do you remember, Dad, when we went to the zoo and had a lovely time ...' She may have been trying to break up the marriage but was also expressing anxiety and insecurity by her behaviour. To her, every sign of affection between the adults was experienced as a stab of pain, a deliberate attempt to ostracize her. Her continual bad behaviour was an attempt to test her worst fear: that nobody wanted her.

'You are not my real mum. I hate you', is a frequent cry of despair hiding anger or jealousy. It may be an expression of having no control over events, or of the child feeling she does not belong to the new family. To the stepmother the 'real mum' can feel as much a part of her family as the actual members. She appears to be the children's secret ally, undermining the functioning of the family like a malevolent ghost. The natural mother, of course, may play no part in this fantasy.

Things will improve once the adults' anger has lost its intensity and there is respect for the child's strong feelings towards her natural mother, who is part of her and is an archive of the details of her life before the divorce. If the natural mother is treated with at least politeness by the new family, she will become a real person and the child will benefit. The alternative, for parents to continue arguing and making unpleasant remarks, is the worst possible experience for the child in the middle.

Sometimes bereft children deal with their problems by stealing, using substitutes to reduce the sense of loss, and maybe to have personal secrets in this new family where there are felt to be many secrets. Material goods have a symbolic value for the child; tangible expressions of being worth something.

Of course, not all stepfamilies have such severe problems. A great number of children develop real affection for their step-parent and believe their life has been better since the divorce.[7] These seem to be children who have not felt a conflict of loyalties between their natural parents, and were given time for the new relationship to develop. The majority want to belong to a stable family, but perhaps have not been made aware that they can contribute to the family happiness themselves; they can give positive messages as well as receiving them, take responsibility for daily chores and contribute to the well-being of the family. But for this to happen it must be appreciated that each will play a different role in the new family depending upon personality, experiences in the first family and relationships in the second. Basically, as for all children, they have needs which should be met.

RELATIONSHIP WITH STEPSIBLINGS

Children in families where other children visit their non-custodial parent and come back loaded with goodies feel an emptiness, for it is the different way in which children feel they are treated which matters. If only one child in the family has a new bike or is allowed to go on holiday with the school or gets preferential treatment, then the other children's self-image, level of depression and behaviour will be affected and, subsequently so will their degree of adjustment, unless parents acknowledge the problem and handle it sympathetically.

Many stepchildren acquire stepsiblings when their parent remarries, children they would not have chosen to spend time with in other circumstances but who will be part of their life – a change not likely to be easy. A child of the new couple may be welcomed, or the reverse. Whatever the situation, it is likely that there will be more children around, all wanting attention and all having to find a position in the new family. Sometimes parents fall over backwards to be nice to the stepchild and, in the process, neglect their own child. Two very successful foster parents, who cared for a number of children, would, instead of having a party for each one on its birthday, take the child on its own to a nearby Happy Eater for a meal; two adults giving undivided attention was luxury indeed.

In a newly-constituted family, any child causing concern is more likely to be helped not as an individual, but within a family context, with a concentration on relationships. Children may need to appreciate that they can belong to more than one family without harm. As in other situations, what seems to matter is the feeling of being 'special'.

LONG-TERM EFFECTS OF DIVORCE

Do children's emotional scars heal because they are resilient, or is the long-term effect one of resignation and cynicism? Although at the time of divorce some children felt important because they had a role in the proceedings as an arbitrator or ally, as adults, many felt cheated out of childhood and had to accept responsibility for their parents as well as themselves. A further anxiety relates to their own ability to sustain close relationships, and especially whether they will be able to make happy marriages. Some remember well the unexpected hardship of being poor and deprived of the things they had been accustomed to. Others express feelings of anger in different ways; they hurt people, break things, damage their own bodies or suffer depression, all of them symptoms arising from their inability to stop what was, for them, the ultimate tragedy of their childhood. Children will be affected by the quality of parenting they received before the divorce and the way it was handled, and obviously not all children are so devastated by their parents' separation. Fortunately, subsequent good experiences can reduce distress for everybody.

CONCLUSION

It is not easy for two united parents to bring up children successfully and it is all the more difficult for one to come to terms with over-whelming feelings and change in lifestyle, while having to care for children who have experienced what is, for them, one of the severest traumas possible – one that has rocked their world to its foundations. At least one parent wanted separation while their children, unless they were involved in violence, wanted unity; two opposing forces which have to be reconciled.

The Children Act 1989 emphasizes parental responsibilities; the children of those who take this seriously are likely to have a good relationship with both parents after divorce and to move freely between them. Providing a safe, caring environment at a time of so much stress can be achieved by co-operation rather than continued conflict. Parents have the task of helping the other parent to do as well as they can for the children, despite their own feelings. An understanding of the children's thoughts, especially their sadness, is another vital ingredient in avoiding possible long-term harm to their self-esteem.

We cannot put Humpty Dumpty together again, but we can do more to ensure that the adverse effects for the children of divorce are minimal.

8 PARENTS: SOCIALIZING AND CONTROL

How parents encourage children to behave in the way they want is not simply a question of framing rules for them to obey; parents' childhood and subsequent personal experiences play a part, as well as their beliefs and the generally accepted values and attitudes of society. The focus of this chapter is what is commonly perceived as the control of children, but which is better thought of as part of the process of socialization.

THE VALUES OF SOCIETY

One of the many myths about families which abound today is that, with some exceptions, they are happy. If there are difficulties, one or both parents are commonly thought to have failed and, because the emphasis is on blame, it is not easy to admit the family is troubled. These attitudes make it hard to reach the best solutions. The reality is that many families are stressed and unhappy and, despite the present emphasis on family values, there is a lack of real support; consequently the difficulties in providing a good environment for children to develop well are likely to increase.

Many parents feel that, despite the plethora of advice, there is neither a basic principle nor a framework for child-rearing which is generally accepted. In these circumstances it is easier to accept the facile denigration by 'experts' of those who have spoken on the subject in the past – Spock in the 60s, Truby King in the 20s – without regard to the times in which they were writing. We may think we do better today and don't make the same mistakes but, nevertheless, we are confused about what to put in the place of these allegedly outdated ideas. There is a danger that this vacuum may be filled by a return to harsher methods of child-rearing embodying physical punishment.

Families do not function in isolation; they both influence and are influenced by the culture in which they live. In Britain today the prevailing philosophy prizes personal success and satisfaction and individual and family happiness to the almost total exclusion of common aims achieved by co-operation. Many people try to bring up conforming children with good academic levels, social skills and self-confidence, to which may be added (especially for boys) the ability to control emotions. Success is equated with high monetary rewards and the material possessions and benefits which money brings: large cars, expensive holidays, luxury housing, as well as better-than-average services in health care and education. Parents understandably want the best for their children as well as for themselves.

The effect on child-rearing is that what is important is not success for group or school, except on the games field, but for the individual and his family. Those who are not successful are thought to have only themselves to blame. Our acquisitive society has little time for those less well endowed with mental or material assets. By implication, we all start from the same point but determination and hard work distinguish the winners.

One concomitant of this kind of thinking is that in striving for success, honesty in all fields is not so highly prized. Respected businessmen are found to have cheated companies of millions of pounds; politicians and civil servants are more blatantly 'economical with the truth' than they were and are less likely to acknowledge mistakes or resign, even if they are accountable. This, of course, is a generalization to which there are many exceptions, but morality is not strongly highlighted and, because the emphasis is on individual success, the ends are often seen as more important than the means. Children cannot escape this cultural pattern.

CHILD-REARING: A HISTORICAL PERSPECTIVE

Given the present uncertainties about how children should be brought up, it is worth briefly considering what happened in the past and whether anything can be learnt from it. Granted that the evidence is scrappy and inadequate, a longer view may help to put matters into perspective and, although it may look like a diversion, it is relevant because the present ways of relating to children are transient; in the next century they will have changed.

To begin with, if a child's relationships are as important as suggested in previous chapters we may wonder how children fared before the idea of showing them affection, once they had passed babyhood, became the accepted pattern. They certainly did not all become delinquent or mentally ill. They seem, generally, to have been treated without the understanding now thought essential, most of the affection and concern shown in diaries being evinced by the child's illness or death. This view is still the subject of debate but there seems to be no reason to project the myth of happy childhood back in time – yet the affection shown to babies may have been adequate to produce later mental health.

Childhood, with the connotation of almost complete dependence, was much shorter and the tasks expected of children were within their competence. Children gained an identity and self-esteem by having at an early age (certainly under ten) the responsibility of work, which in turn led to acceptance beyond the nuclear family in the kin group or locality. The importance of performing useful work probably gave children esteem in the eyes of adults. Many in middle childhood had periods of living away from home, either working in agriculture or in service, being educated (schools and teachers were often far away) or, when they were about fourteen years old, apprentices to a master. At this age they were capable of doing responsible, adult work and in this respect their gradual transition from child to adult was nearly completed (Ben-Amos, 1994).

It is also very difficult to know how children responded emotionally to the omnipresence of death. Religious belief, with its insistence on the vivid reality of heaven or hell, provided a powerful sanction on behaviour for many, inducing both hope and fear and sometimes a resignation amounting to fatalism.

Given how little evidence remains for the history of childhood, it is difficult to discover just how children were reared and how, or to what extent, they formed bonds with others. Many must have had close relationships with siblings. What knowledge we have about those who lived before the beginning of the nineteenth century comes largely from articulate, educated parents who were a minority, although this is changing as a variety of legal documents now being studied give a broader picture. Obviously, warm feelings existed between people in the past but the emphasis on close personal relationships does seem to be a phenomenon of our own time and culture. People are social beings, needing contact with others, and we may surmise that children, brought up at a time when privacy was not considered important, were rarely left alone at home. This must have countered the sense of abandonment that might otherwise be expected.

The changing patterns of child-rearing reflect the different needs and assumptions of society. To give one example, pre-nineteenth century England wanted an obedient workforce which would accept hardships at work; the virtues of honest toil, respect and obedience were therefore primary. With the change to an industrial society there was a need, besides these attributes, for men with educational skills; thus intellectual achievements became increasingly important. Today, the duties of parents include providing educational opportunities for both boys and girls.

Childcare practices are influenced not only by the hoped-for end product – what society wants from its citizens – but also by beliefs about the nature of the child. Some previous generations, believing children were full of mortal sin, thought the duty of parents was to inculcate obedience by breaking the child's will. A good parent was one who vigilantly pursued this task, accepting that physical punishment was necessary to ensure the child's salvation. That vestiges of this still survive is indicated by the acceptability of corporal punishment for the child's own good.

CHILDREN IN SOCIETY TODAY

WORK

Nowadays many people need an added skill on top of their special knowledge and qualifications; that of working in a team. The ability to get on well with colleagues and not be a 'loner', to be assertive but not too aggressive (certainly not passive), and to be able to relate to those in authority without diffidence or brashness are some of the techniques needed. The group is important in this context, but because it includes the element of self-interest, there is no conflict with the emphasis society now puts on individual satisfaction and happiness. Nevertheless, these complexities of working life place greater demands on parenthood which has become more self-conscious. Fortunately, the majority of parents are concerned with the quality their family's life and aim to have reasonable, happy children who grow into successful, well-adjusted adults.

AUTHORITY

One of the most profound changes in recent times has been in attitudes towards authority. People holding positions of power – police, schoolteachers, judges and politicians – do not command the automatic respect they received in the past. Whether or not they have jeopardized their power is open to argument and not our concern here; the effect on the children is. If a policeman apprehends a child for a petty crime, a proportion of parents will blame him, not the child. A head-teacher taking action against blatant disobedience may find himself dealing with irate parents who accuse him of picking on their child. Now that adults no longer present a united front it becomes possible to play off one against another – an enjoyable game, maybe, but not one to create feelings of security in the child.

CHILDCARE

Society collectively has not valued children in the past for their own sake except as cheap labour, but now there is more acceptance that what happens to them influences their adult life. The notion of the family as a stable influence is paraded, although little is actually done to strengthen this stability for society's most vulnerable families. A central problem is the compelling need for many mothers to work. They can be lone parents working to get bare necessities or the family needing two incomes to cover the mortgage. Some women have more personal reasons, related to their profession or personality, for needing to be employed outside the home. All want alternative care for their children, yet its quality varies greatly; lucky indeed is the child in this country who is looked after by one caring person until she goes to school or finds a place in a well-run nursery.

Essentially, the problem of childcare in this context is one of conflicting attitudes: on the one hand is the economic necessity of many women to work, on the other is the meeting of children's needs. There is good evidence that what is crucial is whether the mother is satisfied with her lifestyle.[1] The present compromise provides an inadequate amount of care, some of it of indifferent quality. For older children, too, after-school provision is very difficult to find although here, as with the younger children, there are pockets of excellence.

A variety of successful patterns exists and different options should be available. Evidence from Sweden and elsewhere suggests that care by others, far from being detrimental to development, is beneficial provided it is of high quality. Sadly, many children in England are being left with underpaid, inadequately trained carers who neither give stability nor provide a stimulating enjoyable environment. Care of young children is too important a matter to be left to 'market forces' at minimal cost.

FAMILY DEPRIVATION

It is easy to talk about parent-child values in a middle-class context where they are not affected by inadequate material conditions, but adverse circumstances – notably poverty – make the task vastly more difficult. An inadequate income is likely to affect the level of housing and the health of the family and it can lead to psychological stresses, especially depression, in mothers of young children. Many poor people are isolated and are sometimes further handicapped by their poor education and lack of opportunities. A feeling of being apart from the mainstream of society is far more common than many better-off people realize and makes the task of giving a child a secure base with warm, caring relationships very difficult. As the number of poor families grow, so do the resulting problems.

Providing benign, age-appropriate control is one aspect of parent–child values that is very hard to maintain under the pressure of material deprivation. It is not impossible, though, and those who insist solely on the alleviation of poor circumstances often do injustice to the inner strength and resilience of very poor people, especially mothers, who really do put their children first, emotionally as well as materially. The charge of enforcing middle-class values can be refuted on the grounds that these values cut across class boundaries. The six-year-old, only child of two highly successful media personalities, who was cared for by an uncaring teenage 'nanny' when she wasn't at school, and in despair slashed her wrists, was as deprived as the poorest child in bed-and-breakfast accommodation.

PARENT AND CHILD RELATIONSHIPS

About a decade ago a psychologist watched eighty-five pairs of adults and the same number of child–parent pairs for three minutes each as they walked in streets and shops and stood at bus stops. In that period three-quarters of the adults had some friendly contact with each other. In the child–adult pairs, rather less than half had negative contact (hitting, being told off, ignoring the child when addressed); a similar proportion had no communication and fewer than ten per cent had a positive interaction (Yule, 1985). Yule, the psychologist who made these observations, asked whether parents are so stressed or overburdened that they cannot relate to their children in a friendly way, and she wondered what this sort of rudeness does to a child's curiosity and self-esteem. She thought it related to the low esteem in which mothering is held; there is no joy in doing things which make us feel incompetent. We might ask whether the situation has improved since her survey in 1985 and what the implications for parenting are.

The intention of this chapter is not to increase parents' feeling of guilt, for they are not completely logical, unemotional machines, but people with moods and feelings dealing with others who can be irrational and difficult. It is not disastrous if parents are some-times irritable and impatient, worried and preoccupied, because this is normal and, provided the parent–child relationship is usually warm and joyful, no harm is done. That said, it may be helpful to consider some principles governing successful parenting, so that those bringing up children have a model in mind to which they can approximate.

Many people imagine that the perfect parent for children is one who is always available, kind, patient, reasonable, always puts the child first and is never cross. Ironically, this view might be of value for babies; for children of any other age it is misguided. These paragons of virtue have to hide their own feelings of irritation and can never be bad-tempered or do what they want. They set stand-ards which are maintained at great emotional cost to themselves and are quite impossible for the children to emulate. They may be martyrs who are less than honest in their reactions for fear of upsetting their child with a negative response. The child is con-fused; what does she have to do to get a reaction? She struggles with trying to understand what is right and what is wrong. It is difficult to be angry in such a household, though in some families of this kind the child is the one who is angry on behalf of her saintly parents. Either way she is not learning about making repara-tion and expressing caring feelings after being selfish or difficult.

Other children have to compete with a rival they do not know and cannot see and have no way of knowing why they are unhappy. A sibling may have died and not been mourned completely; as a result the child is a 'replacement' incapable of doing better than the unseen rival. Others can be in competition with a baby who never was, a fantasy-child conceived when the mother was pregnant; very much alive in the mother's thoughts but bearing little relation to her real child who is noisy, demanding, inquisitive and untidy. Perhaps the real baby was the wrong sex (often an important indicator of later difficulty), or had the wrong personality or appearance.

Other parents sometimes do not appreciate the importance of acknowledging their children's individuality and can easily believe that 'he's like his father', is the explanation rather than considering the situation from the child's point of view, or using their own experience as a child to try to understand the message behind the behaviour.

Another aspect of parenting is that there is an optimal time for a child to do new things or meet new challenges and if this is missed there can be difficulties. Andy's mother breast-fed him until he was four in the belief that this was what he needed, whereas the real reason was to meet her needs for a dependent baby. He was deeply distressed when he started school because of separation anxiety and often his caring mother had to fetch her crying child from school.

Highlighting some of the patterns found in families which have problems may give the impression that parents are to blame: this is not the view subscribed to here. Good parenting is not perfect parenting but 'good-enough' parenting. In all the situations described above, the majority of families find a satisfactory solution without outside help. There are many different ways of bringing up children, and because some parents know their own children better than any expert, they are the best people to have this responsibility.

SIBLINGS

It goes without saying that most children are delighted with a new baby and relationships between brothers and sisters can be warm and caring throughout childhood, but this is not always so and can be a great source of unhappiness for some.

Many preschool children have the experience of having a new brother or sister. For some time the child will have been aware of changes in the way she has been handled and, perhaps within three months of the expected birth, will be told formally. The 'Why?' questions will follow and some of them will need honest and careful handling. 'We love you and want another child like you', or: 'It will be a brother or sister for you to play with', are not likely to be as helpful as presenting the change as something which happens to very many children; a normal event with some advantages and some disadvantages.

Obviously, it is not a good idea for the birth to coincide with starting nursery, but to arrange for the child to spend short periods being cared for by other people does make sense. Giving messages about the toddler being extra-valued before the birth will help to lessen the jealous feelings which are usually present, as will letting the older one decide when she wants to move into a bigger bed or when she is prepared to sacrifice some of her toys.

After the birth she sees the baby receiving a great deal of attention and loving care, but has forgotten that she, too was treated similarly at the same age. Her reaction might be to want to taste breast milk or try a feeding bottle again. She will no doubt use diversionary tactics when the baby is being fed. Her feeling of rejection is not one the baby will feel if he remains the youngest in the family because his special position has not been challenged by any newcomer.

Articulate Simon, on seeing his new brother, asked his mother why she wanted a baby when she already had him. Such a feeling, shared by many small children, is not difficult to understand. This is a major change in a child's life, especially for the first-born who has been used to plenty of attention. Ironically, children who have had a great deal of adult time are usually better equipped to accept the newcomer positively.

Jake, at his first meeting with his new baby brother, pretended to be the burglar stealing the jewels (maybe somebody would take this baby away), then changed to being the dustbin-man, so getting rid of the 'rubbish' legitimately. He put his mother's slippers in the bin, followed by the paper in which presents for the new baby had been wrapped. Make-believe, by using symbols, can be wish-fulfilling without the guilt. The fantasies can end as the child wants them to, and positive feelings then have more chance of being expressed.

Some children can cope with an immobile baby but undergo a change of feeling when the new baby breaks the models, scribbles on drawings, bites and pulls hair. 'The baby doesn't understand', is not much help, nor is the parents' acceptance of the destruction without comment. To encourage the toddler to be the big brother or sister for a while and enjoy playing at a much younger level might be an enjoyable experience – especially the smashing games – provided there is time for age-appropriate play when the baby is not around.

Parental reaction will also contribute to sibling rivalry if real or imagined differences are emphasized and the children are perceived as opposites – good/bad; clever/slow; happy/miserable. Such unnecessary labelling will influence the child's picture of herself. 'They are as different as chalk and cheese', is a phrase to be avoided by parents as such comments can become labels. If my brother is so clever or contented, thinks the child, then I must be silly or miserable. In fact, it's all right for both children to be clever or quick, happy or 'good'.

The child who hears her mother telling people how jealous she is of the baby is more likely to have such feelings than the child who is told that later, when the baby gets bigger, it will be able to play but now it takes parents' time and attention and this cannot be helped. The toddler cannot be expected to love the new baby as a matter of course but the relationship might be more positive if it is pointed out that the baby watches the toddler and obviously thinks she is wonderful.

Feelings of concern and anger are likely to be mingled in some degree. Matthew said he did not know why the baby was crying while he was nursing it; he thought no one could see him twisting the baby's foot under the shawl. Once he 'accidentally' rocked the pram too hard and the baby fell out. 'I was only helping', he said, 'it was an accident'. On other occasions he played with the baby, making it laugh, and the relationship was completely harmonious.

At this age, time as a concept is not understood, so the bald statement that one day you will be able to play together is meaningless. The child might think along the lines of: I love the baby but I hate it, too, because it has come between me and Mummy. But I mustn't show too much anger otherwise Mummy won't love me at all. I'll help by fetching the baby's clean nappy. The child thinks nobody will guess what murderous feelings are inside her. Who can be surprised at the bad dreams of children dealing with such a change?

Often children do appear more difficult, miserable or withdrawn, but mothers can contribute to this by being more restrictive and punitive with their first-born, who are not played with as much and receive less attention than previously. A study of children in this situation concluded that it is helpful to talk to the toddler in terms of the new sibling's personality, feelings, wishes and intentions.[2] The authors point out that the experience also has its positive side; the toddlers were found to use their own resources to make developmental advances because parents were not so available.

Some mothers, understandably preoccupied with the new baby, do not have the mental energy to consider the feelings and demands of the toddler. This, then, is a time when fathers can play an important part in developing their relationship with their older child to the benefit of both.

THE INFLUENCE OF THE PARENT'S CHILDHOOD

A parent whose own needs were not met when young will bring early experiences into the present. A mother who knew hunger as a child has difficulty in dealing with her child who is 'faddy' or wastes food. Another who was not allowed to cry could not deal sympathetically with her own crying, distressed child. A father's own parents could not allow any expression of negative behaviour from him, leading to his difficulty in setting appropriate limits. Another father brought up in a children's home without love and understanding deals with his own children by hitting first, then asking questions, because this is how he was brought up and he had never questioned his behaviour. Change comes by being exposed to different, more effective, reflective ways of parenting.

In innumerable ways problems can relate to the unresolved difficulties of the parent's own childhood. The child may be a reminder of an unacceptable part of the parent or of a sibling who aroused jealous emotions. What belongs to the child and what to the parent? Sometimes parents can, in a perverse way, be pleased at what is happening; fathers especially can enjoy having a son with spirit, doing dangerous or daring acts they would have liked to do.

Mike's father was rather different: he gave his son double messages about wanting him to do well at school. Secretly, his son's success made him feel inadequate, so that he constantly chided Mike for not getting top marks while making it impossible for him to do his homework in peace. The unresolved feelings of Chad's father related to a belief that if his family had not come to England when he was a teenager he would have been a doctor; this, then, is what his son must be, so Chad, with average ability, was frequently beaten for failing to do well enough to satisfy his father. Parents using their children to resolve their own unsolved difficulties do them a disservice.[3]

How the past influences the present is illustrated by Maria Brown's story. Maria was finding it difficult to go to school and in a meeting with mother and daughter the counsellor learned that Mrs Brown had had the same problem when she was at school. Mrs Brown giggled as she remembered her own mother writing notes to the school saying she was sick when she was no such thing. The counsellor invited her to say something about her mother and was told that she was a clinging person, very attached first to her own mother, then, after her death, to Mrs Brown: a repeated pattern of difficulties in separation. Mrs Brown, asked how she had felt about this close attachment, erupted angrily as she remembered how much she resented not being free to play out with other girls or go to the Youth Club. She stopped in mid-stream at the thought that Maria might also feel both anger and love. Maria's independence had been forgotten because of her mother's need to feel loved by her daughter. She was pleased that Maria needed her so much but for the first time saw the problem from a different angle. So did Maria.

Another example, with different feelings involved, is that of Mrs Jones who was having a very difficult time with her two-and-a-half-year-old son Paul. Bonding had not been very successful and any warmth in their relationship had gone. Despite her repeated good intentions she had called him stupid and more than once had told him she wished she had never had him. He refused her food, broke his toys, soiled his pants and rarely said anything except 'no'. She was frightened that one day she would lose control and harm him. In the course of an interview with a counsellor she was asked who he reminded her of, and without hesitation she said he was exactly like her brother who was five years older than herself. She was silent for a long time; then tears trickled down her cheeks. When she was able to speak she described graphically how for years she had been bullied mercilessly and lived in tremendous fear of him. She could not express the hate she felt but it was being given expression in her relationship with her little son. She left the interview saddened but relieved, saying she had a lot of things to put right.

WAYS OF CONTROL

A common belief is that children must adapt at all times to parental needs. Parents who hold this opinion may be unable to tolerate their child's reactions to orders: 'If you look at me like that I'll hit you'; 'Don't you dare answer me back'; 'Slam the door as you go out and I'll ...'. A child's angry response may evoke feelings (often sub-sequently denied) which undermine their parents' confidence. The thought might be: don't show me how you feel; your pain, expressed by anger, is unbearable to me.

Parents, fearful that such minor rebellions could develop into serious antisocial behaviour, feel bound to exert control: 'The trouble with free expression is that it leads to spoilt brats and children must be taught right from wrong', is the thinking. The controls they impose, not being related to what has actually happened but to possible future behaviour, are therefore unlikely to be effective. Parents walk a tightrope; those too closely identified with their children will have some difficulty in providing a stable framework of accepted behaviour, while those too distant and unable to empathize with the child are likely to be strict and over-controlling. It is not easy and certainly not an innate skill, and there is no single way to be successful.

So how can parents get children to do what they want in a way which is right for both? How are conflicts between parent and child resolved by methods acceptable to both sides? Basically the question is whether there are general principles which can form guidelines. Different approaches are discussed below, but the way in which children are controlled is possibly the most contentious issue of parenting. What follows will certainly not please everyone.

CONTROL BY THREATS

'If you are naughty nobody will love you'; 'You will make Mummy ill because you are so disobedient'; 'I'll leave you', or, 'I'll have you put away', are fairly common ways of controlling children, but they can evoke basic fears of loneliness and abandonment. It can start when the child is very small and won't leave the shop. 'Mummy's going now and will leave you here'. Attempts to control by inducing feelings of fear cannot fail to be harmful, even if only to a small degree.

Parents may use the desire of older children to be like their peer group. A new kind of difficulty is caused by children wanting the clothes and toys they see advertised, for it is not just a question of having trainers which fit: they must be the right sort with the right name. Alternatively the child says that everyone in the class has a particular toy which was advertised on the television. Not to have one is not simply to be deprived of the article but also to feel isolated from the group, socially disadvantaged, different. What is important is not what sort of person you are but what you own; not your personality but your possessions. This presents the parents with a weapon. They indicate to the child that if she doesn't do what they ask they will not buy what she wants for prestige – important to her enjoyment, and the passport enabling her to belong to a particular group.

Cathy was very keen on swimming, her enthusiasm undiminished by her parents' constant threat that they would not take her to her training session on Friday unless she did what they wanted. This was an effective form of control which they were pleased about, but the price was high. Although the swimming was not directly related to whatever they wanted her to do, the threat built up hidden resentment inside Cathy because she was aware that in this matter they had all the power. What they didn't know was that she regularly helped herself to their money, never taking enough to be missed, but enough for her to feel that she had a secret and was getting her own back.

CONTROL BY DEPRIVATION

This technique leaves no bruises but can cause deep inward scars. The 'pin-down' system, in which children were left in isolation for long periods, is an extreme example of how some children were controlled in a Staffordshire children's home. The basis is 'time out', a technique of behaviour modification where children are isolated from their group until they have calmed down and are ready to be compliant. From personal knowledge I know that children who have been controlled in this way find the experience extremely frightening; bad dreams and further disturbed behaviour can result. The problem which led to the time out is soon forgotten by the child because the isolation is so terrifying. What could be helpful for a child who needs two or three minutes to recover from a frightening feeling of being out of control is turned into something negative and damaging.

Loss of pleasures, sweets, television, pocket money or liberty (to be 'grounded' is the current expression) all deprive children of things they like. A child might well wonder what the link is between the behaviour and the punishment. If a boy has come home late and as a result is forbidden to watch television he may find it difficult to understand the connection, so creating confusion and resentment in his mind.

A different sort of deprivation is to remove a parent's interest and attention. The parent who sulks and refuses to speak to their 'naughty' child is inflicting a punishment of gigantic proportions. To be such a bad child that you are treated as if you were not there can leave deep scars.

For preschool children, being excluded from parental or other relationships is difficult to accept. 'She always plays up when my friends come', is a frequent experience for mothers of young children, though from the child's point of view this can be slightly more tolerable than having to deal with a parent's telephone conversation when the rejection is experienced as complete. This is the time for the child to be extra-demanding – you must come *now*. If this fails, talc can be scattered over the bathroom floor or the baby's clothes put down the loo. The feelings are not new, but increased mobility and imagination mean that the possible responses of the toddler are endless. What the child has lost, albeit temporarily, is the awareness of having some control; when she feels excluded she has lost what little she had.

CONTROL BY HUMILIATION

Sarcasm is a powerful tool which causes humiliation and resentment and often a long-term sense of failure. Even as an adult, an eleven-year-old girl remembered her mother's threat to tell her friends that she wet the bed, a threat she could never forget or forgive. Fancy still doing that – you are a baby. You're the black sheep, the brainless one, a disgrace to the family; you never do what you are told. All these are said so often that the effect on children might seem negligible but, nevertheless, in the long term they undermine self-esteem.

CONTROL BY PAIN

Physical pain or the threat of it is another way of controlling children; its basis is fear. Violence may be uncontrolled or deliberate, and in the latter case is justified by parents on the grounds that the child was warned. 'If you don't do it by the time I count three I will hit you: one, two ...'. Obedience is the result, but at a cost. The child is thinking how to retaliate but at the same time the feeling that she is bad and deserves punishment is confirmed.

If corporal punishment is actually used it conveys the message that aggression solves problems. I do what Mum wants because she will hurt me if I don't, so if I hit my little brother he will have to do what I want. If the aggression is taken outside the family, bullying may result and violence becomes a way of life. Children's pain, anger and sadness may be forgotten but remain within until they, in turn, become parents who hurt and humiliate their own children. They justify their action by believing that such treatment did not harm them and deny the lifelong effects of such humiliation. This superficially valid point of view is only one of the harmful assaults committed on children in the name of discipline.

Already a number of countries (Sweden, Finland, Denmark, Norway and Austria) have banned all physical punishment of children in the belief that those who seriously hurt their children invariably say that the incident started as 'ordinary' but got out of hand. A complete ban, therefore, not only helps to change the climate of opinion about children's rights, but also to reduce the incidence of serious assault. In England at present (1995) corporal punishment can be inflicted on children outside the state system of education and it can be, and is, inflicted in the home. Voluntary bodies such as EPOCH (End Physical Punishment of Children) still have a lot to do to create attitudes which acknowledge that children are persons, not possessions, against whom physical force should not be used.

NO CONTROL

At the opposite end of the spectrum are parents who find it difficult or impossible to set any limits, whose children are perpetually testing boundaries to see how far they can go and who, far from being happy, are anxious and uncontained, often looking for control somewhere.

Tom had parents like this who were almost too kind, not wanting him to be angry with them. 'You are only young once', they would say to justify this inaction, believing that there would be enough unpleasant things he would have to do when he was older, and that childhood should be a happy time. But Tom was by no means happy; without being able to put the thought into words, he perceived that his parents' behaviour met their needs, not his. Their unwillingness to frustrate him in any way resulted in his having no experience of fighting the emotional battles which are part of independence. After tumultuous adolescence he found a very dangerous job, as if to continue the testing, but this time of himself.

Children who are always on the receiving end of kindness do not develop empathy and have great difficulty in considering other people's needs and feelings; they never make the imaginative leap required to share others' emotions. For them adolescence can be difficult as they attempt to solve their emotional problems by demanding material goods, but in this they are unsuccessful; these are not their true needs.

CONTROL IN PRACTICE

YOUNG CHILDREN

Sometimes mothers describe their small babies as 'naughty' because they cry, but this is the only way the baby knows to express discomfort or the need for closeness. It is not possible to spoil a new baby but it is possible not to meet important physical and emotional needs.

If a parent reacts with understanding and empathy to the infant's signals about being uncomfortable or hungry, bored or tired, anxious or fearful as well as those which indicate contentment and pleasure, the infant develops, it is thought, a delusion of power. It is this belief in being able to make good things happen which encourages the growth in self-esteem, independence and creativity.

A slightly older baby also has difficulties because she cannot say what she wants or what is the matter; she has to rely on the understanding of those who care for her. Problems arise if parents do not appreciate her limitations; she has not reached the stage of being able to share, and has no clear memory of what she did yesterday that made people cross. Many of the children who have been killed by their fathers or stepfathers have failed to do something which is completely beyond their ability, as for instance, the baby who was expected to unwrap her own Christmas presents.

Around the age of two is a time of testing and learning what is acceptable behaviour and what is not. Parents who are inconsistent or subject to mood swings may greet with anger the behaviour they found funny yesterday, and this is difficult for the child to sort out. The parent who is shouting angrily but smiling too is a source of confusion for the child.

Until they are aged about three it is thought that children will not be able to appreciate other people's feelings though, of course, there are exceptions. But an understanding that if, for instance, you pull someone's hair it will hurt, generally comes later; it is therefore bewildering for a child who has not reached this stage to have her own hair pulled or arm bitten 'to show her what it's like'.

A mother finds the non-stop demands of an under-five very exhausting and her perception of being a good parent is far from the reality of her situation. Every other mother appears much more patient than she is. This child is making her feel a failure and useless as a parent, especially as 'she is a perfect angel' with everybody else. What is happening? Mother and child are out of step for the time being. The mother may have forgotten that acceptable behaviour can be achieved by subtle distractions and requests rather than orders, using a change in the tone of voice if the issue is important. Parents have to bear in mind the individual differences of their children – some like to be warned that it is nearly time to stop playing, others not. Some respond to the implication that big children clear up toys; little ones don't. But parents are not perfect and they do not always have the patience to take note of these subtleties.

CHILDREN TREATED DIFFERENTLY

Within wide bands the degree of strictness does not matter, but what is certainly damaging is for the children in the same family to be treated differently. If the older one always has to accept that her three-year-old brother is allowed to destroy her drawings, knock down her models, bite and hit her when he is cross, she will develop strategies for getting attention. Among these may be being 'naughty' which, from the child's point of view, may be better than bottling up a sense of unfairness and anger. This is not good child-rearing; the older child feels undervalued and the younger one is not being encouraged to take responsibility for his behaviour and becomes too powerful.

The mother (although equally it could be the father) might be encouraged to understand what is happening. Is she instrumental in repeating the pattern of her own childhood? Is the younger child special because he is the last or because he is perceived by his mother as hers alone, the one who is going to make her feel good about herself as a mother? Sometimes there is a physical likeness or the favoured child is perceived as having the same personality, and sometimes this is the child she would have liked to have been. Similarly, there are as many reasons for an older child being treated as special. Whatever the often unconscious feelings, the parent's belief that there's a special bond makes it difficult to see the child in its own right and thus to set appropriate limits and impose even the slightest discomfort when appropriate.

In families like this the other children are well aware of the situation. They all want to go to the fair: 'You ask', they say to the favoured one, since this will manifestly increase the possibility of a successful outcome. In reality all the children suffer; the indulged child is aware of the power she has over the parents and over the other children who, inevitably, will be blamed for joint unapproved-of behaviour. Similarly, 'If you don't give it to me, I'll tell Mummy', is a powerful threat which often works well, for the other children know that in the end they will lose.

The unfavoured ones may protest but it will be in vain. They become resentful, for if one is favoured the others feel rejected to some degree. They will find other ways of getting attention which may or may not be acceptable to parents, but more sensitive children realise that their best chance of being valued is to give way to the favoured sibling. 'Let him have it', they say, in an attempt to receive some praise for their kind behaviour. All will be tense and show signs of insecurity.

The value of working with whole families is very apparent when one child is treated differently from the others. If, for instance, a parent believes that his or her small acts of spoiling are not noticed, evidence from all the children which reveal the contrary can be a powerful factor in starting the process of change. Some painful rethinking is needed before the situation improves.

CONTROL WITHOUT UNDERMINING SELF-ESTEEM

The parents' task is to find ways of getting essentials done, such as persuading young children to go to bed or get dressed, for instance, without the child losing face. Success is more likely if orders are kept to a minimum and the testing to prove who is in control avoided; there are enough battles which have to be fought without the inessential ones. Negative labels must be removed to avoid their becoming self-fulfilling prophecies. Nevertheless, parents do have a trump card in that their child wants to be loved and valued, but this should never be used overtly.

'I love you but I don't like what you do', is too subtle for small children to comprehend and never helpful; neither is 'You make me upset when you are naughty', for guilt is one of the strongest reasons for misbehaving and this sort of remark merely reinforces such feelings. The last thing the toddler wants is to feel that the people she loves do not understand that the forces which make her angry are too big for her to deal with without some help. But it is right for age-appropriate limits to be set to help the child feels secure – and for the parents to maintain their sanity.

Of course, fear of the consequences – punishment – is one way of setting limits which can be effective in the short term. Children have short memories of events, and if threats become an important part of the relationship, the situation is wearing for parents and undesirable for children because the discipline is external. Better to use children's desire to please rather than sour it by using even a small element of fear in the name of discipline. Better also to use the small child's natural curiosity which makes her easy to distract. Best of all is to reduce the number of confrontations to the minimum by shared activity and mutual enjoyment and by making sure that attention is received for acceptable behaviour far more often than the reverse.

The aim is for the child to want to please, something she learns by having her efforts valued and her behaviour which is not approved of ignored as far as possible. Gradually the child's own conscience becomes more powerful than discipline which is imposed externally.

POSSIBLE GUIDELINES

As children grow and develop, moving through different phases, the adults in charge of them have to change their techniques, basing their behaviour on the stages of development and the unique needs of each child. There are many permutations depending on the individuals involved. No rules, but hard-and-fast guidelines can be put forward. In this context it is worth repeating an important principle – if it's working; fine. If it isn't – try something else.

Respect

The first guideline is that if you want respect from a child, you have to respect the child first. This means being attuned to feelings. The tired child does not really want the crisps or another ride or whatever is being demanded, but rather some understanding that she has had enough for one day. The schoolchild who has been bullied does not want to be told to fight back – in fact, part of respecting the child's feelings is to know when to avoid saying what you have said a hundred times already. More helpful is to talk about what it would be possible for the child to do, such as find some friends, avoid situations which are risky or learn to pretend to be courageous (and contain anxiety) as a preparation for real courage. Such discussion encourages the child to feel that her feelings are not dismissed out of hand and she is not alone with her problem.

Respect implies giving children a message that you think they can cope, you believe in them. All the reassurance in the world will not cancel out the negative remark. However many times Judy was told she was bright, it was her father's comment that she was as 'thick as two planks' when he was helping her with her maths homework which remained with her even into adulthood, undermining her confidence for many years. 'Why did you do that? You are silly', is just as unhelpful. The parent is reacting to what the child thought might happen, rather than a disastrous outcome in her bid towards independence. 'What were you hoping might happen?' is more likely to give a message that the child had a legitimate reason for the behaviour, however misguided.

Respect is not about giving an unending string of praise – 'That's really good'; 'You are clever'; 'I think that's marvellous', and so on. Such phrases, repeated without thought, lose their meaning for the child: there is no differentiation; the picture might be upside down and still get the same response. 'I like that; the colours are really good', gives a message that you have actually looked at it. For a child struggling with, for example, learning to read, to be told: 'I think you have tried very hard' (if the child has), can be encouraging. 'You have been helpful today', is appreciation of what has happened; it is not related to morality and issues of being 'good' or 'bad', and tomorrow might be different.

A contrasting view was that of a father who believed that good behaviour should be the norm and therefore not commented on, while unacceptable behaviour must be followed by punishment. If obedience is the aim then this philosophy might be a way of achieving it, but the child's feelings are ignored and her self-image is not likely to be enhanced.

Parents can become so fearful of disobedience that they forget to comment on approved behaviour, yet if punishment for unacceptable behaviour is relied on then there is the danger of being 'bad' becoming a lifelong label. Consequently, it is better, for example, to give extra pocket money for helpful acts rather than to deduct money for 'naughty' behaviour. In fact, punishment plays little or no part in this way of bringing up children: it will not help them; its only value is that it may help the adult regain control if the situation has got out of hand.

Praise, then, if spontaneous and not mechanical, is helpful but the aim is for the child to be pleased with accomplishing the task, not to gain approbation. Parental attention is the reward. A child who perceives herself as bad, for whatever reason, will find any praise difficult to accept; it does not fit her image of herself. Often interest is what is required, not praise. Nor should non-verbal messages be forgotten; Margaret Harrison's words, that 'a hug is worth a thousand words', contain a powerful truth.

Clear Communication

A second guideline is that parents have to believe in themselves so that when they make a reasonable request they speak quietly in a tone of voice which says that they expect the child to do what they ask. This makes communication clear and the message straightforward: 'You have five minutes to finish your game'; 'When this programme has finished it will be time to go to bed'; 'While you are cleaning your teeth you can be thinking about which story you would like tonight' – these are unequivocal, and are phrased to avoid orders which can be refused. The aim is to reduce confrontation where possible: 'OK, you don't want to put your coat on but I'll put it in the bag in case you feel cold later on.' Another technique is to give choices: 'We have got to buy some bread and some apples but if you would like to spend your pocket money, too, we must go straight away. What do you think?'.

Making restitution may be more appropriate than punishment. 'I know you are sorry for pushing the baby over and making him cry. I wonder if there is something you could do to make him stop?'. That part of the child's feelings which is not sorry can be ignored at this stage in order that she can make things better without losing face.

This approach can be appropriate to a child who is misbehaving. She is giving a message about things not being right, and parents may need to consider whether they should be communicating with the child in a different way. 'You do what I say because I am your Dad', is a threatening statement which may have the desired effect but cannot stop a child thinking that one day she will not be as powerless as she is at present.

Some parents delay responding to misbehaviour until their anger is dominant; at a slightly earlier time they are likely to be more reasonable, and sometimes for the young child the reaction must be immediate. But there is a place for strict limits: 'You are not allowed to throw stones/kick/bite/hurt people/damage property' said in a deliberately firm voice with eye contact, gives a clear message about what behaviour is not allowed without compromise or confusing the issue with threats, punishment or moral comments about being naughty. At other times action is necessary – 'If you don't stop fighting over the television immediately, then I shall turn it off'. Actions, not threats or 'one more chance', must follow, however much the child protests. It can be hard for parents to do what they say because they feel guilty or are fearful of the consequences; some believe that the child will not love them if they set limits, but this is not so.

Sometimes parents forget to listen. Too often, 'having a talk' about misbehaviour is really the parent doing the talking – the child may or may not be listening. 'Stop sulking and say something'. said in an aggressive way, will not make the child feel that there is an opportunity to put over her point of view, nor that it will be considered with respect. Reassurance can also be unhelpful if what is wanted is a discussion of troubling issues.

Giving orders, making threats and negative remarks about the child's failures or lack of skill is one way of relating; a better way is to let the child be in control within reasonable limits. It is her picture so it does not matter if the cows are blue and the fields are pink because it is far more important that she made a choice and it is respected.

Parents might do well to consider what proportion of the orders they give are essential: 'Put your gloves on'; 'Don't run, you'll fall'. It won't be the end of the world if her hands get cold or, provided there is no danger, she goes on running. And are orders being repeated to no effect? Are they expressed clearly? 'I'm tired', should not really mean (for the older child): 'Make me a cup of tea'. Allied with this approach is the necessity of emphasizing the positives. 'Don't touch'; 'Come here'; 'Put it down'; 'Be quiet'; 'Walk by me'; and: 'No, you can't have it', repeatedly endlessly as mother and child walk round the supermarket is demoralizing for both of them.

But communication also involves playing. 'I enjoy playing with you', is a message which makes the child feel special and gives her confidence in herself; the benefits will be long-term.

Sometimes reasoning may be forgotten because adults overlook the child's growing ability to reason herself. 'It isn't naughty to run across the road but it's dangerous. You must hold my hand so that I can keep you safe.' The little girl who told the police that she did not get into the strange man's car because 'Daddy told me to fink, so I finked', expressed something very important. Even quite small children can be encouraged to 'fink' rather than simply to be obedient.

The Child's Point of View

If a child is being difficult, parents need to consider whether something is missing. From the child's viewpoint, either she is being reasonable and it makes sense to her to do what she is doing, or the unconscious reasons for her behaviour are stronger than the possible painful consequences. I know I shall be punished for eating all the biscuits but the pain and emptiness inside me is unbearable at the moment and I must do something about it. This might be her thought but there are other possibilities. What is she thinking and feeling? The parent who gives the child time, one of the important basic needs, is more likely to be able to answer the question. If children are deprived of this and left to their own devices for too many hours in the week they will find a way of protesting. If they are not given opportunities for legitimate stimulation they, with their peers, will find excitement somewhere; if they cannot be helped to find acceptable ways of expressing anger they will destroy what is precious; if they feel unloved their behaviour will be an attempt to deal with the resulting unhappiness. These are just a few of the many situations children face which influence feelings and thus behaviour.

MAKING CHANGES

How can parents be helped to take control when a child dominates the family and their current methods of control are not successful or pleasurable? As a first step parents have to think why this has happened and what has prevented them from giving the child benign limits. It may be that the idea of being both firm and loving is new to them. Or they could be so concerned with discipline that the consequences of controlling a child by even an element of fear were not appreciated. Perhaps the importance of an immediate response, whether approval or disapproval, has not been appreciated. In some discordant families the unacceptable behaviour can be seen as a reaction to the conflicts, a way of survival but also a statement about family loyalty – this is how we behave in our family.

Part of the process of modifying an unsatisfactory family situation involves parents making an often painful examination of their own feelings and relationships. Some can successfully make changes themselves but others benefit from specialist help, for example, from a family therapist who sees the problem in terms of how the family functions, and who teases out its myths and assumptions, its alliances and way of communication. An alternative approach focuses on relationships between family members and will find out these things by another route. In contrast, a psychoanalytical approach might explore the parent's childhood experiences, looking for unresolved conflicts and repeated patterns. Psychiatrists and child psychotherapists are trained to help the child to understand unconscious feelings which affect behaviour, though they also use other techniques. Whatever the method, small changes which are likely to produce successful results can give the family confidence to make bigger changes.

Parents may be helped to understand their children by thinking of what they themselves want from the important people in their lives. However much this varies, some constants will emerge: the desire to be respected, to know that their actions and opinions are valued and people are pleased to be in their company; to have it demonstrated that they matter and they want to be treated in a way which shows warmth; to be comforted and have their confidence boosted when things are difficult. An awareness that these needs are shared by children can help understanding.

In general, when difficulties arise within the family, especially serious ones, parents might do well to consider the six basic needs of children (Chapter 1) to see if any of them have been overlooked.

THE AIM

The real purpose of controlling children has to be borne in mind throughout their growing up. It is to make living easier and more enjoyable for all the family and, in the long term, for the children to grow into successful adults able to live in harmony with themselves and others. It is not about obedience.

9 COUNSELLING CHILDREN – THE PRACTICE

CHILDREN IN FAMILY MEETINGS

Family therapy, a generic phrase incorporating different strategies, has been extensively written about.[1] The varied approaches will not be discussed here; instead, I shall concentrate principally on children in family meetings. It is a personal statement describing one way of working.

Usually parents seek help because a child is behaving in an unacceptable or worrying way. The value of involving all the family members is to provide time and space where everyone can listen to each other, with the emphasis on helping them make changes in order to solve their own problems. The difficulty may relate to how they communicate, but counselling may be needed to alter the emotional distance between people if it is either too close or too far.

A further problem may arise in situations where anger is not expressed, either because it is banned completely or a family member has the monopoly of its expression. Other families don't feel or don't express warmth for each other or one child is not treated with affection and respect. Unresolved past traumas or losses may also be affecting present functioning.

Many other patterns lead families to seek outside help but, in my experience, these are the amongst the most common. Here it is assumed that, however negative a person's behaviour may appear, it hides deep-seated needs for caring relationships and self-esteem; the behaviour is necessary to deal with fundamental fears relating to feeling unloved and inadequate.

Unless the whole family is involved it is all too easy to accept the parents' picture of, for example, 'the boys' or 'the twins' without appreciating that the children have different personalities and experiences. They define themselves in relation to their siblings: 'Mummy loves my sister best but Daddy loves me'; 'Adam is the naughty one in our family'. Even children only a year old are very observant and notice when their sibling is getting special treatment. The competition for parent time and affection is of great significance to them all.

Research shows that children perceive each other and the relationship between them differently (Dunn and Plomin, 1990). If A thinks B is marvellous and they get on well together, it does not necessarily follow that B thinks that A is equally wonderful. In working with families the importance of checking any statement with all the children cannot be over-emphasized.

THE COUNSELLOR AND THE FAMILY

A counsellor (who may be male or female, but here will be referred to as 'he') will be concerned to understand the family's usual way of interacting. He has to be caring and interested but also emotionally outside the family system, otherwise he can become part of it, trapped in its psychological web; a co-worker can help to avoid this happening.

He is an initiator who, merely by being with the family, is communicating something. This must be positive for the family to feel supported and valued. The counsellor, by listening and sharing, is giving a non-verbal message about their being important and deserving his respect for struggling with what is a difficult problem for them. He gives them time to think matters through. In my view he will, in the attempt at clarification, avoid being dogmatic: 'I wonder if you are feeling ...', is better than: 'You are telling me that you ...'. Homilies are never helpful; self-insights by the family or the individual often are.

A useful concept for the counsellor is that of an 'internal supervisor' (Casement, 1985), that is to say he should have the ability to watch himself as well as family members in order to monitor each intervention he makes. The family may try to trap him into being a friend or giving advice; neither is likely to be helpful. They probably have friends and are likely to have had more than enough advice already.

Internal supervision of this kind will increase the counsellor's awareness of what he is avoiding so that, for example, his own unresolved feelings of loss may affect his ability to empathize with a bereaving family; or a recent divorce may cloud feelings when dealing with others' marital difficulties. It will also help him to acknowledge his own fantasies, such as being a good parent to the family and to avoid projecting onto them patterns which belong to his childhood. Most counsellors have these feelings; internal supervision increases awareness of them.

In differing degrees family meetings are concerned with the present, concentrating on the problem the family brings. Here the preferred way of working is to consider the past as throwing light on the present. In my view, to take account of individual psychology is as essential as seeing the person within the family group; the individual's psychological development is, as it were, a vertical line intersecting the horizontal dimension of the family's current situation. As individuals, people are finding the best solution they can, based on their personality and past experience; as family members they are responding to others. Each member of the family is unable to change the way the others react directly, but may change his or her own response. Giving up any behaviour is not easy, especially if it had a purpose in the past and has remained long after the situation has changed.

Therapy is not always successful. This may be because the timing is not right or the difficulties will require a long-term commitment which the family are unwilling to make; sometimes they know, perhaps unconsciously, that their own solution is best at the present time. In other instances failure is related to the personality or approach of the counsellor which does not make family members feel comfortable or hopeful of change. Failures as well as successes are multi-causal.

FAMILY MEETINGS

The physical setting is important. Ideally the chairs – one for each family member plus the counsellor – should be placed in a circle, within which is a low table with paper and felt pens and, if the children are small, a few other carefully chosen toys such as a family of dolls and furniture, animals with fences, and playdough.

At the start the counsellor explains that confidentiality will be respected unless it appears that someone is in danger or they agree to sharing information. It can be helpful if he tells the family what he knows about them, then they know there will be no secrets and the tone of the meetings will be one of shared exploration. The counsellor may be knowledgeable about understanding families, but in many ways this family are the experts when it comes to understanding their particular situation.

The initial contact can be of great significance; the child therefore should be addressed directly. A statement which acknowledges her anxiety because she does not know what to expect in this new situation and may be fearful of the consequences, can be reassuring. She needs to know a number of things: that she has come to a place where children are not labelled as good or naughty but because somebody, such as a parent, is worried about them or they are worried about themselves; that nothing will happen except that people will talk, though children are free to draw or play if they choose; and, if only to reassure her that her ordeal has a limit, the interview will last about an hour.

If it is true, the counsellor should say he will not tell anyone what has taken place, unless a child is in danger. Finally the aim of the meeting should be stated in general terms. For instance, the counsellor might say that the purpose of the meeting is to help everyone feel happier or get on better together and this usually means everyone having to look at some uncomfortable feelings about events which have happened or are happening now.

In a family meeting the children are given as much respect and as much opportunity to express their views as the parents are. At one time it was thought that very young children detracted from the main purpose of a meeting but in fact they are very useful members of the group, their drawings or play often mirroring what is happening between the adults.

This type of family work is often painful and difficult, but at times it can also be enjoyable, for family and counsellor alike.

SOME QUESTIONS

A number of questions will help understanding. It might be best to start with a fairly general one which can be answered by the family in whichever way they choose. The counsellor could start by saying: 'Tell me about your family'. He will be listening to the factual information, always clarifying obscure points but at the same time noting who has started talking, who is listening, who is anxious, what the atmosphere in the room is like. The greatest help to understanding is awareness of one's own feelings: this person who has not spoken yet is making me feel angry; why? During this initial exploration the counsellor will be making comments to indicate interest and occasionally asking other family members to confirm, deny or elaborate. It is important that everyone contributes to this discussion. On one occasion, after the parents had talked at some length about their family, a six-year-old said: 'You haven't told the lady you don't ever speak to each other at home'.

Another important early question, asked of everyone in turn, may be: 'Why are you here?' It can be revealing to hear what the children have been told because it indicates the degree of openness in the family. Children might have expected to be criticized by the counsellor or threatened in some way: 'The man's going to put you in a Home'. Some will be confused. One Child and Family clinic shared the waiting room with a dentist. The interview had lasted about ten minutes when a small child asked when his teeth were going to be looked at.

Some subsidiary questions may be relevant provided the children are not made to feel inadequate because they cannot think of an answer: how does it affect you; who is most worried, what do you think might make things better, what would you like changed? 'Who does he/she remind you of?', is another question which might lead to a discussion of some of the family myths, such as, for example, that all the bad attributes come from one side of the family. It may transpire that the family believe one event caused their difficulty. 'It all started when we moved house'; 'There wasn't a problem until the car accident'. These explanations could easily be part of the problem, perhaps the trigger which, when pulled, started the war, but other factors will have kept it going. Just like people, families can become emotionally 'stuck' and might need some help to move forward.

NON-VERBAL CLUES

Much can be learnt about how the family relate to each other from non-verbal clues. Who is sitting next to whom? Who comforts the baby, who is irritated by the crying? Are the toddlers reacting timidly or by racing around, attracting attention in their anxiety at being in a new situation? Is one child showing concern about the parents' responses, another clinging to a parent or a third behaving in a younger way than her age would suggest? Some, to hide anxiety, giggle uncontrollably; which parent attempts to control them may be significant.

As the discussion continues, the child or children will be playing as well as listening. Often the play indicates that the children are listening intensely. As one mother shares her distress at her childhood rejection, her small son draws a picture of a small boat with a person in it shouting: 'Help, help', while a large liner steams away. Both he and his mother are the person in the boat, abandoned in a sea of tears.

Do the children share, or quarrel, and if so, who intervenes? Is there cooperation or rivalry? Do they want adult praise and interest or can they use their own resources? Is there a child who distracts when a parent is becoming upset or angry, one who is more adept at picking up adult feelings than the others? Is one left out? Which child relates to one parent, which to the other? Is there more mess and destruction than normal? Much can be learnt about the family by watching.

HELPING THE CHILD TO TRUST

Many children have learnt by experience that adults cannot be trusted; secrets might be told, confidential information used later to undermine the child, or important information trivialized. In such circumstances trusting the counsellor will take some time.

The key elements in encouraging trust are honesty and respect. Honesty means never compromising what is said to protect family members, although at times it is appropriate to avoid answering questions if an answer would be unhelpful at that particular moment. White lies akin to reassurance are usually not helpful.

Respect means listening with empathy rather than asking questions or giving advice. It means staying with the child's pain without offering the usual placatory comments and it means always allowing the child to decide the areas that he is not prepared to discuss at that time. A gentle approach is essential, well-expressed in the phrase: 'Without tenderness the noise of our talking does harm' (Hobson, 1985).

Occasionally, parents come to the meeting determined to recite a list of misdemeanours – sometimes written down – and are oblivious to the child's distress while the attack is in progress. It may be necessary to give a positive connotation to the 'bad' behaviour being reported; the counsellor may wonder aloud if there is an explanation other than disobedience. Could the child be trying to distract the family from a painful situation, or is she attempting by her actions to unite the parents so that they will not be cross with each other? Maybe the parents could also think of some possibilities? Maybe the children could help?

It might also be helpful to hear what punishment has been tried and to ascertain that this solution has not worked; otherwise they would not need outside intervention. To react differently would mean considering what purpose the behaviour serves for the family and whether they could react in a different way. This sort of response can indicate to the child that the counsellor is not concerned to think up bigger and better punishments as there might be a positive reason for the behaviour and some understanding of the underlying reasons would lead to a more positive solution for her.

AIMS AND ENDINGS

Usually there will be a series of meetings. The overriding purpose, after establishing what is causing the family distress, is to help its members change the way in which they interact with each other. The family may see the problem in terms of a symptom such as Johnny's stealing, or Sally's reluctance to go to school, or whatever, but there is some understanding that this is the tip of the iceberg; an indication that all is not well.

It is important to get a full picture of the present problem. What actually happens? If Johnny is stealing: When did it start? What does he take? Is he alone or with a group? What does he do with what he has stolen? Does he try to hide the evidence or not? Do other people steal in the family? Could the stealing be related to something missing in his life? Is this symptom especially important for this family? The counsellor cannot presume to know because there are many reasons. By musing aloud, rather than asking direct questions, the counsellor will learn many of the answers without asking. To label the child or attribute the difficulties to one cause is simplistic. When the problem has been discussed the family will be in a position to state what they want from counselling. What are their goals? How can they be achieved?

The end of the contact is as important as the beginning. A contract for a specific period of time can be helpful for some families and when it ends, the work should be assessed. This was the problem which brought them for family counselling and this is the point they have reached now. Perhaps the symptoms of unhappiness are seen differently or there has been a change in relationships. The ways they are interacting may be freer, with more warmth and respect, or the structure has altered and the myths have been exposed. Whatever the changes, if the family have gained in confidence and feel they can solve their own difficulties in the future, then the work will have been worthwhile. But to repeat, this is often difficult, stressful work and there are families who, for many different reasons, do not change.

FAMILY DYNAMICS – SOME POSSIBLE PATTERNS

Ways of communicating will become evident in family meetings. All too often, families with difficulties do not communicate a sense of value to each other or have forgotten how to express warm feelings; compassion has been forgotten. Repeated angry 'put-down' comments reduce the self-esteem of everyone, adults and children alike.

Indications about the structure of the family will also be picked up. One parent may be dominant, whereas in some families the symptom has been allowed to control them all: for example, they cannot go out together because one child upsets everybody by misbehaving, or another refuses to go to bed and so effectively stops the parents having any privacy.

Often when the family is in the room it is difficult to identify the one said to have the problem, for this can be either the child who is emotionally robust and protesting about what is happening, or the one who is outside a destructive family complex. Also, children will respond differently to the same event depending on their personalities.

Sometimes a family is emotionally split with children on one side and the parents on the other, or a male parent and female child against a female parent and a male child; sometimes all the males are lined up against all the females. If there is, say, only one female (the mother) in a family of males, she can be marginalized. Where the members of the family sit in relation to one another in the interview sometimes gives pointers to their divisions, but what is relevant is how ingrained these are in the family structure and whether the pattern is constant.

A family member with a monopoly of expressing a particular emotion may have the effect of silencing the children, but at some cost. If Dad is always angry and aggressive, the children learn that it is better to keep their own anger in check.

Sometimes the core relationship is not between the parents but between a child and a parent. All the family members will be containing anger in such a situation; the too-powerful child does not know where the limits are, is less secure than she should be and therefore angry that no one can control her. The other children will feel rejection and anger because they are not the special one. The other parent feels devalued, while the offending one can be angry with him or herself because of a vague awareness that this is not the best way to be a parent. The price paid by the family for this parent being reassured, or flattered, by one child is very high.

Children rejected by one or more members of a family can soon be picked out when all meet together. Problems of rejection have been discussed earlier (Chapter 5); here it will suffice to say that if one child is rejected and becomes the scapegoat for the family she is in a different position from those in families where all the children are rejected or emotionally deprived in some way. She can be the repository of all the 'badness' in the family, freeing the others from blame and disapproval. The roots of the problem are likely to be buried deep in the family pathology, past or present, leaving her no alternative but to behave like her label and be 'bad'. Such a pattern becomes apparent in family meetings. Other children are well aware of the situation, though parents may not be; they don't realize that their tone of voice depends on which child they are addressing.

Fortunately, children in such families are subjected to influences at school and in other relationships which help to counter the negative effect of treating one child differently from its siblings; fortunately, too, children are resilient.

Non-verbal clues can indicate the same pattern. A home visit to a family revealed five photographs of the daughter in the sitting room and none of the son. It was explained that he did not take a very good photograph .... Subsequently it transpired that he was born after a stillbirth; a replacement who could never rival the untested claims of the dead baby. He had to fail, and as all children tend to behave like the labels first put on them by their parents, he did so, and was a cause for concern.

Often parents say: 'We've tried everything. We've punished him and we've been kind and understanding but nothing seems to work'. The unspoken meaning of this might be: we are not going to let you succeed, either. The counsellor will be concerned to understand what the symptoms mean to the family and why have they reached the point, albeit with some ambivalence, of wanting things to change. 'He's been doing it for years, but we think his younger brother will copy him soon.' So why is it all right for the older son to behave in a certain way and not the younger? What would happen if the behaviour stopped? Perhaps the older one would be ignored completely, and is making a statement about his fear of rejection.

SECRETS

In family work, what is not said can be indicative of what is wrong. Many possibilities can account for this behaviour, including an emotion such as jealousy or a taboo on anger which then has to find other more indirect outlets. Often such avoidance relates to a family secret, such as the child's being illegitimate or having a father who is not the person that cares for him. It may be the death of a sibling in the past; there are many other reasons for not sharing important information.

Counsellors have to differentiate between what is secret and what is private. It is not helpful for children to be burdened with every adult secret but it is necessary to share, at the right time and in an empathic way, secrets which have a bearing on the child's image of herself. When Amy was born her identical twin died. The baby was never properly mourned and as the years passed the parents were too distressed to tell Amy what had happened. She unconsciously knew that something was missing, something unexplained. Her symptom of wandering off when she was eight years old could be seen as a search for the unknown. Her parents asked for a private meeting to tell the counsellor about this but were refused. They were told that if the secret concerned their daughter and they had reached the point where they needed to talk about it, it might be right to share it with her. With support and encouragement they did this and for the first time, joined by Amy, cried unreservedly for the daughter they had lost. Amid the sadness there was relief that the secret no longer formed a barrier between parents and child.

A thirteen-year-old boy called Freddie also felt like this; he was so preoccupied about his sexual identity that his progress at school was seriously affected. He could not share his feelings with his family because he knew that his parents had opposing views and would react in different ways, leading to a row between them; better, he thought, to remain silent and to try to deal with his worries himself, thereby keeping the peace. A family meeting provided a safe place where he could share his worrying secret.

A symptom highlighting the fact that something is not right in the family often relates to either the marital relationship or the unmet needs of the child. It is inappropriate to discuss marital difficulties in a family meeting except to help the parents understand how the stress between them affects the child's development. Sometimes it is their perception of parenting which is a problem, not their basic relationship. Glen's mother described herself as a perfectionist, some-one who wanted her house kept beautifully clean and tidy. His father resented this and subtly undermined her, joining forces with Glen whose brashness did not successfully hide his low esteem. Boundaries were not being respected. Some compromises, relating to co-opera-tion and support rather than conflict and disparagement in their role as parents, were necessary before the situation improved.

CHILDREN WHO PROTECT THEIR PARENTS

Many children, aware of a parent's vulnerability, protect them from feelings of inadequacy and distress; this, and many other patterns of family interaction, are exposed by seeing all family members together.

Which needs of the child are not being met is a question the counsellor must always have in mind. Too often, even the most caring parents do not realize the effect of events on their child. Wendy's teachers were concerned about the decline in her work noted soon after her maternal grandmother died. 'Of course she is not depressed', said her mother, 'she is always laughing, she is the lively one, and anyway we are a family who keep our feelings to ourselves.' Wendy, in fact, had given herself the task of keeping her mother's depression at bay but in doing so she had to deny her own feelings of deep sadness. At school she was daydreaming and unable to concentrate. The need to mourn her grandmother was pervasive and secret, but had to be denied in the interests of family stability.

The degree of dependence thought right for each child may be a source of stress. Some older children feel they are not allowed to be themselves and they have no space around them. They may feel safe in their close relationship with one parent but they can also feel both angry, because of the restrictions imposed on them, and anxious about the image of the external world that such closeness engenders: 'I don't think you will enjoy the party but of course you can go if you want to.' The message to the child is that she will not be robust enough to manage without her parent. For other children the parents' wish to encourage their independence makes them feel unwanted and uncared for. To achieve the right balance – and it changes accordingly to the child's maturity – is not easy for parents.

In many situations parents cannot bear their child's pain and are unable to admit that it exists. The child, in colluding in this, protects the parents from their own confusion, distress or failure. For example, parents will deny that a child is jealous of the new baby who has stopped her from having all the parental attention. To acknowledge the feeling sensitively, which would help the child, is very difficult for some people because it means being aware of their own unacceptable feelings of jealousy when they were young. Better to pretend jealousy does not exist.

In exposing these sorts of patterns, family meetings can enable parents to see problems differently and to experience them, not as their child's attempt to hurt but as a message that something is wrong or missing. What is important is that their child is showing by her behaviour that she has not given up hope of things improving. The family will have many strengths; such meetings give them a second chance to use them and go some way to fulfilling everyone's need for closeness and to be valued for their own sake.

THE INFLUENCE OF PARENTS' CHILDHOOD

Other than the human desire to care for the small and vulnerable, parents have no innate knowledge of being parents but bring to the role many different experiences, specially those relating to how they were cared for when they were small. Parents who have not had good-enough parenting are likely to find being a parent more difficult than those who have experienced a loving, stable family, but it is quite wrong to believe that a bad beginning will necessarily result in the pattern being repeated. For some it will, but others, on their journey to adulthood, have the ability to acquire warm relationships and learn from others different ways of managing their difficulties.

The counsellor is often the catalyst enabling unacceptable feelings to be explored safely. They may have been attributed to another family member as a way of denying their influence or they may, especially if the feelings are related to the member's own parents, be attributed to the counsellor. For example, some will reject any suggestion that the counsellor makes because that is how they dealt with their own parents; others complain of not being told what to do. Children will have fantasies, often based on wishful thinking, or may experience the counsellor as intrusive. He will have to separate those feelings which belong to the family from his own.

It is not unusual for families to ask whether they will harm the counsellor, believing their own feeling of badness will affect him. 'Are we the worst family you have dealt with?', they ask. 'Will you be overwhelmed by us?'. That is to say: 'Are we really too awful and undeserving of your time and attention?'. For the counsellor to deny the statement will not help them but may give him some clues about the problem: Who has been overwhelmed in the past? Who did the overwhelming? And why have they got such a poor image of themselves?

An individual's internal make-up is likely to include unresolved experiences from the past, or some important emotional problems that have not been worked out. These basic feelings are usually related to a lack of belief in their own worth or a sense of failure in certain crucial areas of emotional life, thereby resulting in a deep rooted fear of being rejected or abandoned, unloved or unlovable. For others the fundamental fear of loneliness or of being alone, and sometimes the anxiety, or despair about being powerless cannot be faced.

These feelings of worthlessness, powerlessness and the fear of rejection have to be denied, and a number of ways are used to do so. One is the belief that it is better to attack first; another is to retreat into silence. Placating behaviour is in others' armoury, and there is a host of other strategies. All can be seen as useful ways of surviving but the basic, feared emotion will surface in some way. In family meetings the exploration of an individual's deep feelings is not relevant unless it influences family functioning; the focus is not on psychotherapy.

SUMMARY

A problem can be looked at from an emotional standpoint, the emphasis being on understanding feelings and past experiences which influence current behaviour. Alternatively, a more objective approach places the focus on the present problems and relationships, looking at ways in which behaviour and family functioning can change. These two different approaches can be seen in opposition to each other but in family meetings can be complementary, with great effect.

COUNSELLING INDIVIDUAL CHILDREN

A child may sometimes need individual help. This may be provided by a psychologist, quite often in a school setting. A few see a child psychiatrist or psychotherapist who is concerned with the child's inner world, especially her infant experience.[2] For present purposes what is described as counselling is a general term encompassing a number of different approaches. Here the focus is on the environment of the child, present and past, embracing feelings and relationships.

Play

Since children express themselves more easily through play rather than with words, toys are necessary in working with them. What follows is different from play therapy because it is focused mainly, though not exclusively, on the child's present feelings. The aims include: to provide a safe place where a child can share fears and anxieties; help her accept traumas and unwanted experiences; share her feelings of sadness and loss, or be helped to find more acceptable ways of solving problems. It provides a setting where, in play, the child can safely identify with the powerful person and change the ending of the play sequence in such a way that nobody is harmed and anxiety is reduced. Some children benefit from a more psychotherapeutic approach than that described here.

The Interview: Equipment

The choice of toys varies with each counsellor; I suggest that a small selection from the following list should be available, some of which have already been referred to as useful in working with families: drawing equipment, playdough and sellotape; a family of dolls and dolls' furniture including a bath and lavatory; fences and animals both domestic and wild, including some which are powerful – especially crocodiles – but also vulnerable little mice or small furry animals; other toys might include vehicles such as ambulances, fire engines and police cars, a doll with a dummy and a cot and blanket, and possibly two toy telephones and puppets. A big cushion and one or two soft toys which can be safely hit – or cuddled – can be important. Only a few well-chosen toys are desirable for each child. What toys the counsellor provides will depend upon his individual choice, though of course the child must be absolutely free to choose from what is available without direction.

I also have Erik, a very soft, colourful, 22 cm tall doll who came from Germany, and who, although he has big ears, cannot tell anyone what he hears because he does not speak English. He wears a large hat which cannot be removed and under which secrets can be kept safely. Small children are willing to tell Erik about their worries and dreams which they would not tell me directly.

The Setting

One or two basic rules have to be laid down as the need arises; the child will not be allowed to damage herself, the counsellor or the equipment, and toys have to stay in the room, save in exceptional circumstances. One incident will demonstrate the importance of flexibility in this regard. When a counsellor was about to take sick leave for six weeks, she allowed a six-year-old boy to take home a toy of his choice. He chose a small postman carrying a large letter – a symbolic link with the clinic; it remained on his mantelpiece, untouched except by him, for the whole time. At his session immediately after the break the first thing he said was that he had brought the postman back.

The child's feeling of being contained will be enhanced if interviews take place in the same room at the same time of day. It should be free from evidence that other children have been there, such as their drawings on the wall or photographs; she will have enough problems without adding material for jealous fantasies. Privacy and confidentiality go without saying and it is usually better, once the sessions have started, not to have contact with the parents unless the child is present and hears what is said. Sometimes this is not possible or desirable; then the child must have a categorical assurance that what takes place in the sessions will not be discussed without her agreement.

THE COUNSELLOR AND THE CHILD

So much for the framework; what of the counsellor? Because of their need to be special to somebody, children can be adept at focusing on the non-professional part of the counsellor who, in their imagination, is their good parent. This fantasy is never helpful because it cannot be realized and will lead to another rejection, thus adding to difficulties between child and true parent. The work is with the child's feelings, and they will be accessible only if she feels safe with whoever is trying to understand the symbolism she is using.

Attempts at understanding do not always succeed and a sign of progress may be when the child tells the counsellor he has not understood. This type of work is very different from talking to a child and requires more sensitive listening which cannot be done in other contexts. This basic technique of 'reflective listening'[3] involves the therapist following the child's lead and giving a running commentary on what is happening and what feelings are being expressed in the play.

Praise is not relevant. Normally children need to be praised for their efforts and achievements but this is inappropriate in counselling. Rewards come from an inner feeling of success which boosts the child's confidence. A long time ago this was brought home to me very dramatically: a positive comment about a boy's drawing was followed by a long look, then, making eye contact throughout, he deliberately tore it into small pieces and put them under the rug. His belief that nothing about him was good had not been picked up.

It goes without saying that blame is equally irrelevant. Neither is it helpful to express anger on behalf of the child; such expression of the therapist's feelings are a distraction. It is certainly not concerned with moral training, giving advice or making suggestions. None of these can be reconciled with accepting the child as she is.

Finally, the pace of the interview is important and should avoid making the child feel under pressure, a point usefully made by Axline (1969).

LEARNING TO TRUST

It goes without saying that in work with families, the counsellor gaining the child's trust is fundamental to the work. Some testing by the child therefore, may be necessary. 'I dunno', is one strategy, another silence. When the counsellor's concern is believed, trust can begin. Anger may also be around: 'only nutters come and see people like you'. Other children are destructive and rude in their attempt to find out if they will be rejected again. It may be a new experience to be accepted no matter what behaviour is being displayed and will be some time before such children can enjoy having one adult's undivided attention despite the distress which often accompanies the work.

Children use sessions in different ways. Many take a long time before they are safe enough to face feelings and conflicts which they have had to bury deep in their psyche. For others it is an opportunity to share their unconscious feeling of hate as a result of their needs, especially that of being loved, not being met. Depressed and anxious children, angry and aggressive children – all carrying a burden of fear – can be greatly relieved at finding someone who is aware of these terrible feelings and who is not overwhelmed by the intensity of their pain.

Often it is helpful for the children to have their 'naughty' behaviour redefined. Chris, who had a number of obsessional symptoms, was quite determined not to share his anxieties because they were 'private' and adults weren't to be trusted. Only when the counsellor said that he did not see Chris as naughty but as a boy carrying a great weight of anxiety and anger around with him did he feel that somebody has understood a little of his inner anguish, and he decided to risk trusting the counsellor with some of his secrets.

SHELLS

In therapeutic play something quite neutral, called 'a third thing' by Clare Winnicott,[4] is valuable. Shells can serve this purpose, though other small objects such as buttons or stones could be used.

The child is presented with a blank piece of A4 paper and about twenty shells of different sizes, shapes and colours. She is asked which one is herself and this is placed on the paper. Shells to represent other members of her family and other significant people follow. Together the child and counsellor look at the result. The counsellor may need to make an observation to help the child understand the purpose of the play: 'I see you and Daddy are close together'. At this point some children might want to modify the arrangement as they consider family relationships, moving the shells until they are satisfied they have truthfully presented the picture as they see it.

As they consider the result, both child and counsellor make comments. One child used the black cockle-shell to represent himself because, he explained, it is different from the others and he is the odd one out in his family. Another child pounced on the joined halves of the same shell: 'That's definitely my sister', she said. 'Its big mouth – she can't keep anything to herself.'

Gemma, nearly ten, had two younger sisters aged six and four. She used the smallest shell for herself because, she explained, she felt small and the point on the shell was important. It stood for her attacking, angry self, necessary for her survival. In the centre of the finished arrangement was a space. The counsellor said that she wondered about this. 'Oh, that must be the dead baby', said Gemma, with tears in her eyes. The baby had died five years before but the grieving had not been completed. Of greater significance to Gemma was the changed relationships. She moved the shells to show how it had been before the tragedy when she had felt loved and cared for. Afterwards, the second daughter had taken her place, as she was close enough in age to be a substitute baby for her mother. A third daughter, born fifteen months later, became 'Daddy's girl'. Gemma, full of sadness, had lost her special position with both parents. Her feeling of being unwanted had persisted for many years, causing her to feel increasingly isolated and angry, the hate for the sister who had ousted her knowing no bounds.

Seven-year-old Jamie arranged the shells to represent his present family – mother, step-father and two step-children at the top, with himself in the middle of the page, nearest to his mother. On the bottom half was his father and his paternal grandparents, with his father nearest to him. The difficulties of belonging to two families was patently obvious. What was equally obvious was how important his paternal family was to him despite very infrequent visits; all three of them were indicated by the three biggest available shells.

Another boy arranged three large shells which represented himself and his father and mother in a triangle, with his sisters, shown by small shells, some distance away. His father had left the family nearly two years ago and lived 200 miles away, but, nevertheless, this sad little boy demonstrated very clearly his longing for a united family and his inability to accept the separation.

A brother and sister were asked to depict their family; working jointly and with a lot of discussion, they arrived at a consensus. Looking at the result they were surprised at how close the family members were to each other, forcing them to modify their previous picture of themselves as a divided family who related to each other in a hostile way.

Colour, shape, size and position: all can open doors for the counsellor into an unhappy child's inner turmoil; for the child the shells can be a symbolic way of facing what is troubling her and, by giving the feelings tangible expression, help her to have some control.

SILENCES

Silences are important and have a number of different meanings, and while they are taking place the counsellor has to concentrate very hard on the child and attempt to understand what she is thinking. For some, the inner pain is too great to be expressed in words; for others it can be a defiant act, a demonstration of power. But silence is often an expression of anger. After a Christmas break, a normally talkative ten-year-old spent a session in silence. The counsellor, judging only from the top of the child's bowed head, offered the interpretation that his anger concerned the gap in the sessions and it might be too damaging if he let even a little of it out: there was no response and the silence continued. The only fleeting eye contact was at the end of the session when the counsellor said: 'I'll see you again next week'. At his next session the child bounced into the room saying that now he was OK. His wordless hostility had been accepted, therefore he felt accepted. For other children, the experience of not having to share feelings is of value; they are respected and are in charge. To be with somebody, yet alone, feels good.

Silence can be about the child giving the counsellor the experience which she has had repeatedly – that of being shut out and rejected; a 'no-person', as one child expressed it. Equally it can be a message about survival, the child feeling that she needs time to absorb what is happening. Questions are not helpful in this situation, for, as has been said, if you ask a question you only get an answer. In fact asking questions is rarely helpful. It has been rather well put that the only question which can properly be asked is: 'Would you like to tell me about it?' (Axline, 1969).

SYMBOLISM

It is important that the child should instigate the play, although she may want the counsellor to help. Sometimes a child's question needs a direct answer, not an interpretation. How much longer have we got? Have you got a ruler? At other times it is important to clarify an issue. 'I wish I were dead', says the child. 'It sounds as if you feel you have nothing to look forward to', says the counsellor. The remark encourages the child who, until now, has received the response 'Don't be so silly'. By far the majority of his comments attempt to reflect what the child is feeling, usually repeating what has been said or indicating that he is trying to understand.

Play conveys various symbolic messages, the most prevalent being the child's feeling of emptiness or badness. Confusion, fears for the future, fears of being abandoned or lost are often present too. Sometimes play is used to express anger at feeling powerless. All children express these feelings in some degree; it is emotionally healthy to do so. In the disturbed child, though, they are more obsessive and have an intensity about what is being expressed. At other times the message is about being 'stuck'. A boy of ten draws a badge and writes on it 'I am eight'. Clearly the age of eight is significant; something bad happened to him then, or the last two years have been stressful and have to be wiped out.

Stephanie had parents who wanted her to be perfect, not allowing her to express any negative feelings. Her play was very contained at first but as she became more trusting the animals were thrown round the room, paper was torn, and everything was tipped onto the floor; by the end of the session the room would be in chaos. Meanwhile, another counsellor helped her parents to accept some healthy expression of anger and encouraged them at the same time to give her some feelings of success. As Stephanie's inner world became more contained she ended each session by clearing up some of the mess, and after about three months the family no longer needed any more help with this problem.

Insecure Children

The deprived child often focuses on food and never having enough. She may prepare lovely meals, then punish someone or something because they are being greedy. One ten-year-old repeatedly made great banquets with playdough, but before the greedy piglet could eat anything at all a huge rocket came flying through the sky destroying everything, including the little pig.

Deep-seated fears about loss and abandonment are expressed, too, in drawings about a deep, deep sea populated with dangerous sharks who swallow small defenceless fish. The fantasies of a deprived child contain a great deal of violence; sometimes the whole world and all the future is annihilated in an angry, hopeless scene of destruction.

The feeling, common to insecure children, of not being 'held' is indicated in many ways. Lost animals, people falling, things falling apart, water falling or floods are some of them. Alternatively, things will be joined together obsessively. A little girl who could not accept her parents' separation used masses of sellotape to join things together. Nothing in her world was stable. One session she spent making little balls of plasticine and repeatedly let them trickle though her fingers. Nothing was contained; nothing was safe.

One way in which the child can avoid painful experiences is to talk about fantasies that bear no relation to her own feelings. They may refer to cartoons or something seen on television. The counsellor must see them as what they are and, recognising that they will not advance understanding directly, accept them as an important mode of communication.

Rick spent time drawing a football game, reflecting an age-appropriate interest, and in the same session drew a room full of large, scary spiders – an outwardly ordinary ten-year-old containing a frightening inner world.

Drawings

Understanding the symbolism of a child's drawing is a special skill. What is important is the overall feeling. Is the whole page used? What is missing? What about colours? No straightforward relationship exists between the drawing and its meaning. For one child, red means blood, for another, warmth, and for a third, anger. A series of drawings is much more revealing than one on its own, and to say: 'Tell me about your drawing', is not always helpful, whereas: 'I wonder who lives in that house', might open the door. Drawings should always be kept because this is a message about valuing the child and what the child produces, as well as providing continuity to the sessions. Many children are interested in the changes expressed in what they produce over a period of time and will verbalize the feelings associated with past work.

The depressed child may draw bleak or black pictures, often including dead trees. Houses have an empty space in the middle and are devoid of people, although children who have become skilful at covering up their own distress to protect their parents will draw happy, smiling faces until they realize that it is acceptable to share their true feelings.

The fantasy of the pre-adolescent child who draws ghosts may be an expression of the fear of reprisal for her 'bad' thoughts, which are quite probably related to jealous feelings or anger at not being valued. If her parents knew her thoughts, she fears, there would be no chance of being special.

Animals

Using the animals, Tony made up a story of a black sheep falling down a cliff and no one hearing its cries. 'That little lamb sounds upset and lonely', says the counsellor. Tony agrees and says he is feeling afraid, too, because he is standing on a very small ledge and if he fell from such a great height there would be nothing left of him. They discuss the lamb's feelings about disappearing for ever and then wonder if anything could save him. At no time does the lamb consciously become Tony and all the time it is Tony's story – he is in control. He repeats the play sequence many times until he finds an ending which is satisfactory to him.

The way children use the same toy varies greatly. Duncan used the eagle as a savage bird devouring the peaceful animals. In fantasy he was in control; an unusual situation for him. For timid, non-speaking Jill, the eagle represented freedom to fly everywhere in the room; for some brief moments she allowed herself to throw off the tight bands which constricted her while she soared into the sky.

Lions may guard the house or more often be used to express anger, but the crocodile with its sharp teeth and gaping mouth is perhaps the most frequently-used wild animal. It can stand for mothers who fail to be, in Donald Winnicott's words,[5] the 'ordinary devoted mother'; or the greedy child, or the powerful forces that could swallow you whole and make you disappear for ever. In contrast, the kangaroo with its pouch and the camel with its two humps usually represent the good, caring mother. Fences are useful in understanding the child's messages about her fear of fragmentation but can also symbolize keeping the uncontrolled wild parts of her inner world safely enclosed.

Four-year-old Ray used the rhino in his play. He had been very close to his mother when she was pregnant, and after the pregnancy ended in a miscarriage, he believed that he was in some way responsible. The rhino who represented himself had a monkey fastened to its back with playdough, and for a number of sessions he played with these two animals, indicating that he was trying to accept the fact that although there was no baby, he had not killed it.

Dolls

The families of dolls and their furniture are used in many different ways. Some children arrange the furniture in separate areas, one person in each part, as a reflection of both an uncommunicating family and the fragmentation inside the child. Three-year-old Kathryn repeatedly gave the dolls baths and was upset when she could not remove the doll's clothes. Her curiosity about adult relationships and her anxiety about her own sexuality were very evident from the way she played. Philip, in contrast, was dealing with the arrival of a much wanted little sister – wanted by his parents, that is. The baby doll was usually hidden in a cupboard or behind a chair by the end of the session.

Summary

These are a few of the innumerable symbols used in play sessions. Each play sequence has a different meaning and will only be understood in relation to unresolved conflicts and unmet needs for security. Many of the examples may be seen as manifestations of negative feelings but, at the same time, in each child there is a tremendous drive towards growth and health which will also be symbolically expressed in therapy. Everyone, of whatever age, wants to be loved and be lovable, to be seen as worthwhile and capable, and to belong somewhere. Disturbance occurs when the child finds unacceptable ways of meeting needs. Counselling, by providing a safe place for the exploration of feelings, can help her to find more acceptable solutions.

NOTES

INTRODUCTION

1. This is not a universally held view. See Stone L. (1981, p. 225), '... the link between the adult personality traits and the infantile experience remains no more than an interesting speculation.'

1 NEEDS OF CHILDREN

1. Kagan (1984, p. 111). Trauma, the arrival of a sibling, the quality of maternal affection or the authoritarian behaviour of a father – these are the kinds of event which move a child toward certain choices and away from others. In Kagan's words, 'once a choice is made, the child will resist being detracted [distracted] from that path.'

2. Kellmer Pringle's book *The Needs of Children* (1975) is still essential reading on this subject. She identified four main areas of need: love and security; new experiences; responsibility; praise and recognition. I accept the basic premise of this important book, but have changed the emphasis to some degree as a result of the growth in understanding of a child's relationships within the family.

3. J. and E. Newson (1976, p. 444) This basic need is summed up succinctly: '... the developing personality needs to know that to someone it matters more than other children; that someone will go to unreasonable lengths ... for its sake'.

4. J. and E. Newson (1976, p. 441). The parental task is seen as one of socializing children and the authors suggest parents make a bargain with them: in return for acceptable sociable behaviour outside the home, sanctuary will be preserved within it as the place where the child can revert to her more uncontrolled, primitive self in a babyish way which is respected by the parent.

2 ANXIETY AND FEARS

1. In a comparatively quiet area – the Isle of Wight – nearly 7 per cent of ten- and eleven-year-olds were found disturbed enough to cause significant interference in their ordinary lives (Rutter *et al.* 1970). In an inner London borough the figure was twice as high. More than twenty years on, in far more stressful social conditions, the incidence of such behaviour is likely to be even greater. A striking finding of the research was the length of time the symptoms had persisted; most had been apparent when the children were aged seven and eight.

2. Fraiberg (1959), an American writer, suggested that a baby can experience the need for sucking as an unbearable tension in the mouth.

3. Berger (1985), Graham *et al.* (1973) and Richards and Bernal (1974) were all concerned with the effect of the child's personality on behaviour.

4. Strategies for dealing with the problem are discussed by Douglas and Richman (1984). Jaques (1987) includes it among other emotional problems she considers. Daws (1989) believes that babies are extremely perceptive of parents' anxiety and stress, especially between them: fear about separation, she thinks, may also be at the hear of sleep difficulties.

5. Richman and Lansdown (1988) found that 45 per cent of boys and 31 per cent of girls wet regularly at the age of three and 20 per cent of all children at the age of four.

6. Marjorie Boxall (1976) advocated schools' giving children the experience of early dependency which they missed when they were babies. This is valuable preventative work and still highly effective for vulnerable children. See Iszatt (1994) for an up-to-date evaluation of Nurture Groups in Enfield.

7. Fraser (1973). In Belfast, during or immediately after a stressful event, the expression of acute anxiety could take bizarre forms such as excessive shaking, laughing for no apparent reason or uncontrollable weeping. Symptoms after the event included regressive behaviour, especially clinging, because the need for the presence of trusting adults is very strong. Following a different kind of disaster – that of Aberfan in 1966, when 116 children were killed – sleeping difficulties, nervousness, bed-wetting and emotional instability were the most prominent symptoms reported by children.

   The reactions Fraser described occur in other traumatic situations. Ways of lessening the effects of the traumas are also discussed.

3 SAD CHILDREN

1. Harris Hendriks, Black and Kaplan (1993). The authors believe that it is important for the child to be interviewed within a few days of the event and be helped to remember every detail by playing, drawing or talking about what happened. This puts the trauma outside the child and is necessary before the process of mourning can start.

2. Perkins and Morris (1991). The death of a mother is very sensitively illustrated and shows that it is possible to share the grieving with very young children. It also demonstrates how important a sensitive school can be.

4 CONDUCT DISORDERS

1. Rutter, M., Harrington, R., Quinton, D. and Pickles, A. (1991). 'Adult outcome of depressive and conduct disorders in childhood', referred to in *Young Minds*, October 1991.

2. West and Farrington (1973). The conclusion to emerge from the Cambridge Longitudinal Study was that harsh discipline at eight years of age was the strongest predictor of later violent delinquent behaviour, and a better indicator than aggressive behaviour at that age. Farrington repeated the interviews with 411 of the boys when they were adult and identified six risk factors discernible when the were children: teachers identifying those who were troublesome; low income of the parents; a court conviction before the child was ten; poor child-rearing with harsh and erratic discipline; low intelligence and attainments obvious by ten years of age, and being regarded by peers as daring at eight years of age.

   Unsatisfactory family relationships and discord are undoubtedly important too, but other influences, both antisocial and benign, come from outside the family and should not be dismissed. The child's peer group, his neighbourhood, the attitude of teachers or police to him are just some of these influences. The interaction between all these factors is highly complex.

3. Dockar-Drysdale (1968). For seriously deprived children in therapy a useful division is between unintegrated and integrated children, a process which, for most children, takes place somewhere at the end of the first year. Unintegrated children are unable to use symbols or to think in words; neither do they have the tools to sort out experiences, to understand and share. If these insecure children are not helped they will become destructive at school, irresponsible and unable to show remorse.

4. The findings of a Department of Education survey on bullying in schools (compiled by Professor Peter Smith, 1994) involved 7000 pupils, and found 27 per cent of primary-school children and 10 per cent of secondary-school pupils were victims. The long-term effects are serious for both the bullied and bullies. A pack of information is available to schools (October 1994).

5. Childline (1990, 1991). 8000 of the children who engaged in conversation were studied in more depth. More girls than boys rang; the majority between the ages of eleven and thirteen. The belief that boys should deal with bullying themselves may have stopped some of them from phoning. Girls were more likely to have fallen out with a friend, who subsequently bullied her; boys are bullied if they 'tell' or do not conform in some way. More than half were bullied by children of the same age. These were remarkable revelations.

6. Kolko & Kazdin (1991). 133 parents of firesetters aged six to thirteen were interviewed. The authors identified children as having high curiosity or high anger; if both were present there was greater behaviour dysfunction and more risk of fireraising.

7. Yule (1979). An analysis of 2000 stories written by eight- and nine-year-olds in Melbourne. The children's themes related to the need for food or its symbolic equivalent, security, competence and warm relationships. She concludes: 'We must look more critically at what our society teaches children in the first seven years at home and school and make them less destructive.'

8. Berrueta-Clement et al. (eds) (1984). The High/Scope Foundation, in Ypsilanti, Michigan, is concerned with preschool education. This research was based on a sample of more than 120 potentially slow learners of low IQ. An important element of the High/Scope programme is that parents are involved and there is a high teacher–pupil ratio. Children are encouraged to plan their own activities in a fairly structured environment and to report on what they have done at the end of the day. They are learning to think logically and to take responsibility.

   At present, only a small percentage of three- and four-year-olds benefit from this type of preschool education in Britain. The principles on which the approach is based, without prejudice to the work of those with a different philosophy, might usefully find application in many nursery schools, nurseries and family centres.

9. Poor reading skills and their relation to conduct disorder have been discussed by a number of writers, including Rutter and Yule (1976) and Pringle, Butler and Davie (1966) (p.777), who, referring to the NCB cohort, conclude: 'The incidence of maladjustment at the age of seven

was four times higher among poor readers than among the rest of the cohort.'

10. Kenneth Clarke and John Major quoted in David Rose 'The Messy Truth About Britain's Violent Youth', *Observer*, 28 February 1993.

6   PHYSICAL AND SEXUAL ABUSE

1. Hobbs and Wynne (1986) 'We have become aware of more cases of anal abuse than any other form of sexual abuse in very young children of both sexes'.

7   DIVORCE AND CHILDREN

1. Wallerstein & Kelly (1980). Although this study was begun more than twenty years ago it is still important. The aim was to explore the feelings of the 131 children and assess the effect of divorce on them five years later. The initial period they found profoundly stressful but the effect diminished by the end of the first year, girls recovering faster than boys. A transitional period of two or three years followed, at the end of which some families, but by no means all, had succeeded in making a happy home. The children's experience before the divorce and what had taken the place of the failed marriage were significant.

2. Mitchell (1987, p. 143). Children from fifty families were interviewed. They wanted more information and most wanted their parents together, whatever the conflict. They wanted to talk about the divorce, and seeing both their parents was important. Only young children might blame themselves.

3. Parkinson (1987). Chapter 5 summarizes a variety of conciliation schemes.

4. I am indebted to Mr Brian Smith of the St Albans Civil Unit for the basic idea of a ladder to express changes in thought.

5. Rowlands (1980). The author maintains that activities ought to be geared to the children's interest and be age-appropriate. Younger children appreciate routine, and ritualistic anger in the form of play-fights or other battles can be helpful. He argues that children judge parents in their own terms and whether they show warmth and concern; whether they are fun and interesting, reliable and honest. They do not want to be drawn into adult differences, to have their loyalty strained, or to hear the other parent criticized. They need both parents to understand that

their bad behaviour is an expression of stress and that their changing attitudes are related to developing maturity. Rowlands also points out the pleasures such a relationship can bring, despite the difficulties.

6. Smith, D. (1990). A sensitive examination of stepmothers; the conflicts and confusions of the role exacerbated by society's attitudes to step-mothering. Nevertheless, she does indicate ways in which the experience can be pleasurable and satisfying.

    De'Ath and Slater, (eds) (1992), a more recent stepfamily publica-tion, is a useful summary for parents.

7. Ferri (1984). Using data from the NCB cohort, this study found that the majority of children in stepfamilies enjoyed satisfactory relationships and made good educational progress. Some of the boys were not quite so successful but the differences from girls were not great.

8   PARENTS, SOCIALIZING AND CONTROL

1. Dunn (1988). Discussing the effect on young children when women are working, bringing up children and running a home, Dunn writes: 'Our research brought out one fact clearly. Whether children have a good or bad childhood depends on how satisfied the mother is with her life, *not* on whether she works or not. The children of satisfied working mothers do very well, as do those of satisfied mothers who are at home. The children of mothers who are unhappy or frustrated, whether at home or at work, are more likely to have problems.'

2. Dunn and Plomin (1990). This is a seminal book which discusses why children in the same family are so different, suggesting that it is the different experiences which are important, rather than what is shared. The authors found that those who receive more negative treatment from their siblings than their siblings receive from them suffer poor self-esteem and are less well adjusted.

    Two other important findings are that a child can expect to receive less attention following the birth of a sibling and that children are very sensitive to how their parents treat their siblings.

3. Miller, A. (1987a, 1987b, 1990). Alice Miller has written a number of books in which she relates childhood traumas to adult destructiveness.

9   COUNSELLING FAMILIES AND CHILDREN

1. Barker (1992). This is one of many general books concerned with differ-ent schools of family therapy. Zilbach (1986) is more relevant here.

Cattanach (1992) is also useful, and for brief therapy see Cade and O'Hanlon (1993).

2. The theories of Melanie Klein (1970), Anna Freud (1966) and Donald Winnicott – see Davis and Wallbridge (1981) – often provide a theoretical basis, though non-directive techniques based on the work of Carl Rogers (1951, reprinted 1976) are also widely used in work with children. See also Jennings, S. (1993).

3. McMahon (1992) gives many different examples of therapy with children using 'reflective listening'. Axline (1964, reprinted 1988) is an important book which gives a sensitive, in-depth description using this technique.

4. Clare Winnicott (1968, p. 70). '... a third thing, which unites us, but which at the same time keeps us safely apart because it does not involve direct exchange between us.'

5. In Davis and Wallbridge (1981) pp. 125-30.

BIBLIOGRAPHY

Place of publication is London unless otherwise indicated.

Axline, V. (1964) *Dibs In Search of Self,* Pelican.
—— (1947) *Play Therapy,* Churchill Livingstone.
Barker, P. (1992) *Basic Family Therapy,* 3rd edn, Oxford: Blackwell.
Barker, W. (1994) 'The Child Development Programme', *Young Minds* Newsletter 19 September.
Ben-Amos, I. K. (1994) *Adolescence and Youth in Early Modern England,* Yale, Ct.
Berger, M. (1985) *Temperament and Individual Differences,* in Rutter, M. and Hersov, L. (eds) *Child and Adolescent Psychiatry* 2nd edn, Oxford: Blackwell.
Berrueta-Clement, J. R. *et al.* (1984) *Changed Lives,* Monograph of the High/Scope Research Foundation no. 8, Ypsilanti: High/Scope.
Bowlby, J. (1973) *Attachment and Loss,* vol. II: *Separation: Anxiety and Anger,* Penguin.
Boxall, M. (1976) 'The Nurture Group in the Primary School', *Therapeutic Education,* 2 (4).
Butler-Sloss, Lord Justice E. (1988) *Report of the Inquiry into Child Abuse in Cleveland,* HMSO.
Cade, B. and O'Hanlon, W. H. (1993) *A Brief Guide to Brief Therapy,* New York: Norton.
Campbell, B. (1988) *Unofficial Secrets,* Virago.
Casement, P. (1985) *On Learning from the Patient,* Tavistock.
Cattanach, A. (1992) *Play Therapy with Abused Children,* Kingsley.
Childline (1990, 1991) Annual Reports.
Children Act (1989), HMSO.
Christopherson, J. (1989) 'Sex Rings', in Hollow, S. A. and Armstrong, H. (eds) *Working with Sexually Abused Boys,* N.C.B.
Dale, P. *et al.* (1986) *Dangerous Families: Assessment and Treatment of Child Abuse,* Tavistock.
Davis, M. and Wallbridge, D. (1981) *Boundary and Space: an Introduction to the Work of D.W. Winnicott,* New York: Brunner/Mazel.
Daws, D. (1989) *Through the Night: Helping Parents and Sleepless Infants,* Free Association Books.

De'Ath, E. and Slater, D. (1992) *Parenting Threads*, National Step-family Association.

Department of Health (1993) *The Rights of the Child: A Guide to the UN Convention*, DoH/Children's Rights Development Unit.

Dockar-Drysdale, B. (1968) *Therapy in Child Care*, Longman.

Douglas, J. and Richman, N. (1984) *My Child won't Sleep*. Penguin.

Dunn, J. (1988) 'A Double Act', *New Society*, 5 February.

—— and Plomin, R. (1990) *Separate Lives: Why Siblings are so Different*, New York: Basic.

Ferri, E. (1984) *Stepchildren: a National Study*, National Foundation for Educational Research/Nelson.

Fraiberg, S. H. (1959) *The Magic Years*, Macmillan/Scribners.

Fraser, M. (1973) *Children in Conflict*, Secker and Warburg.

Freud, A. (1966) *Normality and Pathology in Childhood*, Hogarth.

Graham, P. *et al.* (1973) 'Temperamental Characteristics as predictors of behavior disorders in Children', *American Journal of Orthopsychiatry* 43:328-39.

Harris Hendriks, J., Black, D. and Kaplan, T. (1993) *When Father Kills Mother: Guiding Children through Trauma and Grief*, Routledge.

Hobbs, C. J. and Wynne, J. M. (1986) 'Buggery in Childhood – a Common Syndrome of Child Abuse', *Lancet*, vol. ii, 4 October.

Hobson, R. F. (1985) *Forms of Feeling*, Tavistock/Routledge.

Hoghughi, M. (1988) *Treating Problem Children*, Sage.

Iszatt, J. (1994) 'Nurture Groups as an Early Intervention Model', *Young Minds* Newsletter 17.

Jaques, P. (1987) *Understanding Children's Problems*, Unwin.

Jennings, S. (1993) *Play Therapy with Children*, Oxford: Blackwell.

Kagan, J. (1984) *The Nature of the Child*, New York: Basic.

Kahn, J. H., Nursten, J. P. and Carroll, H. C. (1981), *Unwillingly to School*, 3rd edn, Oxford: Pergamon.

Klein, M. (1952) 'Some Theoretical Conclusions Regarding the Emotional Life of the Infant'; and 'On Observing the Behaviour of Young Infants', both in *Developments in Psycho-Analysis*, 2nd edn, Hogarth (1970).

Kolko, D. J. and Kazdin, A. E. (1991) 'Motives of Childhood Fire-setters', *Journal of Child Psychology and Psychiatry*, 32:535.

Lynch, M. A. and Roberts, L. (1982) *Consequences of Child Abuse*, Academic Press.

McMahon, L. (1992) *The Handbook of Play Therapy*, Routledge.

Miller, A. (1987a) *For Your Own Good*, Virago.

—— (1987b) *The Drama of being a Child*, Virago.

—— (1990) *The Untouched Key*, Virago.

Mitchell, A. (1987) 'Children's Experience of Divorce', *Children and Society*, 1 (2).

Newson, J. and H. E. (1976) *Seven Year Old in the Home Environment*, Pelican.

Ney, P. G. (1986) 'Child Abuse: a Study of the Child's Perspective', *Child Abuse and Neglect*, 10:511–18.

Parkinson, L. (1987) *Separation, Divorce and Families*, Macmillan.

Perkins, G. and Morris, L. (1991) *Remembering Mum*, A. & C. Black.

Pringle, M. K. (1975) *The Needs of Children*, Hutchinson.

—— et al. (1996) *11,000 Seven-Year-Olds*, Longman/NCB.

Richards, M. and Bernal, J. (1974) 'Why some babies don't sleep', *New Society*, 27:509-11.

Richman, N. and Lansdown, R. (eds) (1988) *Problems of Pre-School Children*, Chichester: Wiley.

Rogers, C. (1951) *Client-Centred Therapy*, Constable (1976).

Rollinson, R. (1993) 'Report of a Symposium on Violence and Young Minds' *Young Minds* Newsletter 16, p.11.

Rowlands, P. (1980) *Saturday Parent*, Allen and Unwin.

Rutter, M. (1971) 'Parent–Child Separation: Psychological effects on the children', *Journal of Child Psychology and Psychiatry* 12 (12).

—— (1991) 'Services for Children with Emotional Disorders: Needs Accomplishments and Future Developments', *Young Minds* Newsletter 9.

—— (1992) *Developing Minds*, Penguin.

Rutter, M., Harrington, R., Quinton, D. and Pickles, A. (1991) 'Adult outcome of depressive and conduct disorders in childhood', Paper presented to SRCD Symposium, Seattle, Washington.

Rutter, M., Tizard, J. and Whitmore, K. (1970) *Education, Health and Behaviour*, Longman.

Rutter, M. and Yule, V. (1976) 'Reading Difficulties', in Rutter, M. and Hersov, L. (eds) *Child Psychiatry*, Oxford: Blackwell Scientific Publications.

Seligman, M. E. P. and Peterson, C. (1986) 'A Learned Helplessness Perspective on Childhood Depression: Theory and Research', in Rutter, M., Izard, C. E. and Read, P. B., *Depression in Young People: Developmental and Clinical Perspectives*, New York: Guilford.

Smith, D. (1990) *Step-mothering*, Hemel Hempstead: Harvester Wheatsheaf.

Smith, P. (1994) *Bullying: Don't Suffer in Silence*, Department of Education Survey, HMSO.

Stone, L. (1981) *The Past and the Present*, Routledge and Kegan Paul.

Tattum, D. P. and Lane, D. A. (eds) (1989) *Bullying in Schools*, Stoke-on-Trent: Trentham.

Thomas, A., Birch, H. G. and Chess, S. (1968) *Temperament and Behaviour Disorders in Children*, New York University Press.

Trowell, J. and Castle, R. (1981) 'Treating Troubled Children', *Child Abuse and Neglect* 5:187-92.

Wallerstein, J. S. and Kelly, J. B. (1980) *Surviving the Breakup*, New York: Basic.

West, D. J. and Farrington, D. P. (1973) *Who Becomes Delinquent?* Heinemann.

Winnicott, D. W. (1958) 'Transitional Objects and Transitional Phenomena', in *Through Paediatrics and Psycho-Analysis*, Tavistock.

Winnicott, C. (1968) 'Communicating with Children', in Tod, R. J. N. (ed.) *Disturbed Children*, Longman.

Wolkind, S. and Rutter, M. (1985) 'Separation, Loss and Family Relationships', in Rutter, M. and Hersov, L. (eds) *Child and Adolescence Psychiatry*, 2nd edn, Oxford: Blackwell.

Yule, V. (ed.) (1979) *What Happens to Children: the Origins of Violence*, Angus and Robertson, Australia.

—— (1985) 'Why are parents tough on children?', *New Society*, 27 September.

Zilbach, J. J. (1986) *Young Children in Family Therapy*, New York: Brunner/Mazel.

INDEX

abandonment *see* separation
abuse *see* emotional abuse; physical
   abuse; sexual abuse; verbal
   abuse
adolescent children, reaction to
   divorce 103
age-appropriateness
   of independence 158
   of parental control 128, 139
   of parental responses 68
   of responsiblities 10, 74, 75-6
   and unrealistic expectations 87
aggression
   in fantasies 59-60
   and masculinity 65
   reaction to physical abuse 83
   to hide anxiety 28, 46, 48-9
alienation
   and physical neglect 78
   of poverty 64
anger
   at divorce 100
   and conduct disorder 47
   and depression 35
   expression of 27-8, 67, 166, 167
   fear of 15
   in grieving 42
   turned inwards 7, 27, 83, 97
anxiety
   at divorce 100
   in babies 13, 14
   in boys 28
   and conduct disorder 46-7
   develops from specific fears
      12-13

anxiety *continued*
   and the family 26-9
   from external events 25-6
   from outside family 29
   and school refusal 30-2
   symptoms of 21-3
   in young children 15, 16-21
   see also fears
arson 58, 174n
attention
   behaviour modification
      techniques and 23, 143-4
   see also time
Austria, physical punishment
   banned 138
authority, attitudes to 78, 126-7

babies
   and bereavement 39
   crying 13-14
   fear of being abandoned 13,
      172n
   meeting needs of 139
   physical abuse of 82
   sexual abuse of 96
   sleep problems 14
bedwetting and soiling 22-3, 172n
behaviour
   anti-social 60-1
   bizarre 97
   'nuisance' 46, 47, 62
   see also conduct disorder;
      regressive behaviour
bereavement
   adult reactions to 38, 39